Praise for
Full Circle Health

Appreciating the cyclical nature of women's bodies is the key to unlocking the "mysteries" of our health. Detailed charting is an invaluable tool for achieving a deeper understanding of symptoms and patterns, often yielding insights missed by conventional medical practice. Full Circle Health is an accessible guide for all women to help them begin this empowering journey.

Rebecca Cohen, M.D., Obstetrician, Holistic Women's Health specialist

For anyone who wants to have a deeper connection to themselves or a way to commit to changes in their health and well-being, Full Circle Health is a must-have.

I first became aware of the cyclical nature of my body and mind through Lucy's book Moon Time. This book takes that knowledge to a new level of awareness. It is a hugely helpful and practical toolbox for anyone wanting to dive deeper into themselves or just increase their awareness on a day-to-day basis.

As always with Lucy H. Pearce, it is a gorgeous book to read and very easy to use. I am enjoying the ritual of waking up and filling in my daily pages which has resulted in my journaling regularly again for the first time in many years. This book is exactly what I was looking for and everything I needed.

Mary Tighe, Doula (CD)DONA, GentleBirth instructor, DoulaCare Ireland, BirthingMamas.ie

Another amazing book and useful tool by Lucy H. Pearce. Charting was easy to do as the explanation of how to use the book was very clear to me. I appreciate how it covered healing topics in a succinct manner so a reader gets the idea (if they have no experience in that particular area, for example, moon cycles) nicely planting seeds, which invite readers to learn more in this area. I will be recommending Full Circle Health to clients working to heal digestive issues and food intolerances, yoga students, menstrual and fertility health clients, PTSD suffers, abuse victims, and pregnant-postpartum-nursing mommas… to name a few.

Paula Youmell, RN, Wise Woman Nurse®

Full Circle Health is a book that is truly going to help me identify pain triggers, moods, creativity and so much more. I'm a huge advocate for self-care but usually neglect myself. Full Circle Health gives me the opportunity and a reason to sit down quietly and think about how I'm feeling, and document it. I'm now putting my health first, and that is a pretty big step for me. I'm looking forward to being able to identify my pain triggers, when they happen and how long for, to allow better care from my consultant. From tracking moods and mental wellbeing, through to tracking menstrual cycle or chronic illness, Full Circle Health is adaptable to each person's individual needs and I have never seen anything else like it available.

Tamsin Hopkins, EcoFluffyMama.com, Winner 2017 UK Blog Awards (Green & Eco)

Please note *Full Circle Health* reflects the personal experiences of the author. The information provided is intended to complement, not replace, the advice of your own doctor or other health care professional, whom you should always consult about your individual needs and any symptoms that may require diagnosis or medical attention and before starting or stopping any medication or starting any new course of treatment, exercise regime or diet.

Published by Womancraft Publishing, 2017
www.womancraftpublishing.com

ISBN 978-1-910559-22-2

Cover design, internal illustrations and layout by Lucent Word, www.lucentword.com

Cover art 'Keep a Loving Heart, Mandala' © Elspeth McLean
Artist photograph © Tegan Clark

Womancraft Publishing is committed to sharing powerful new women's voices, through a collaborative publishing process. We are proud to midwife this work, however the story, the experiences and the words are the author's alone. A percentage of Womancraft Publishing profits are invested back into the environment reforesting the tropics (via TreeSisters) and forward into the community: providing books for girls in developing countries, and affordable libraries for red tents and women's groups around the world.

Full Circle Health

integrated health charting for women

Lucy H. Pearce

WOMANCRAFT PUBLISHING

Also by Lucy H. Pearce

Full Circle Health: 3-month charting journal (Womancraft Publishing, 2017)

Burning Woman (Womancraft Publishing, 2016)

Moon Time: harness the ever-changing energy of your menstrual cycle (Womancraft Publishing, 2015)

The Rainbow Way: cultivating creativity in the midst of motherhood (Soul Rocks, 2013)

Moods of Motherhood: the inner journey of mothering (Womancraft Publishing, 2014)

Reaching for the Moon: a girl's guide to her cycles (Womancraft Publishing, 2015)

Contributor to:

We'Moon Diary – La Luna (Mother Tongue Ink, 2018)

Celebrating Seasons of the Goddess (Mago Books, 2017)

If Women Rose Rooted: a journey to authenticity and belonging
 – Sharon Blackie (September Publishing, 2016)

She Rises: how goddess feminism, activism, and spirituality? Volume 2 (Mago Books, 2016)

Wild + Precious: the best of Wild Sister magazine – Jen Saunders (Wild Sister, 2014)

Tiny Buddha's Guide to Loving Yourself – Lori Deschene (Hay House, 2013)

Roots: where food comes from, and where it takes us (BlogHer, 2013)

Earth Pathways Diary (2013, 2014, 2017, 2018)

Musings on Mothering: an anthology of art, poetry and prose – Teika Bellamy
 (Mother's Milk Books, 2012)

Note to Self: the secret to becoming your own best friend – Jo MacDonald (2012)

Contents

Acknowledgements

Over the years I have picked up tools from many women in the quest to better understand my health. I want to fully acknowledge how important their work and guidance have been in my life and in the creation of the concept of *Full Circle Health*.

Firstly, Christiane Northrup whose book *Women's Bodies, Women's Wisdom* I have read almost every year for two decades, whose compassionate and fierce advocacy for women's health seeded my own work.

My understanding of women's health has been shaped by many ground-breaking menstrual educators, especially Jane Hardwicke Collings' powerful Shamanic Midwifery work (now known as Shamanic Womancraft), as well as the work of Alexandra Pope, Jane Bennett, Penelope Shuttle, Rachael Hertogs, Lisa Lister and Miranda Gray.

I have been cycle-tracking since my teens, long before cycle-tracking apps were even a possibility. In my early twenties I learned fertility charting from a practitioner and Toni Weschler's classic book, *Taking Charge of Your Fertility*. For the past seven years I have logged my cycle against the moon in my diary. Favourites include *We'Moon*, *Earth Pathways Diary*, both of which I am honoured to have contributed to, and now our own *Moon Dreams* charting diary by Starr Meneely.

In my personal struggles to put my own physical and mental health experiences into words and images, I have been deeply influenced by the work of Barbara Ann Brennan, especially her book *Hands of Light* and the mood tracker from Dr Liz Miller's book *Mood Mapping*.

The biggest influence on the format of this book was author and creator of the Shining Academy, Leonie Dawson. Her Life and Biz Planners have been instrumental to my personal and business growth over the last few years and they showed me how powerful workbooks can be in moving from feeling to action. It was she who shared a spreadsheet-based habit tracker which I loved the idea of, but quickly fell out of the habit of using. Years of experimenting with screen-based, versus paper-based creativity have shown me that some sort of magic happens when I put pen to paper. The act of physically writing and drawing helps to start the 'flow' – the creative/healing process – in a way that logging habits on a computer does not.

Creative thanks also go to Elspeth McLean, whose art I have loved for many years, and which speaks deeply to the spirit of this book. I am so deeply honoured to use it on the cover. And to Jennifer Berezan whose song "Returning" on the *Yoga Woman* album and Mari Boine's *Idjagiedas* album carried me through this project so gently as I listened to them on loop.

To my dearest husband, Patrick, of Lucent Word, who once again up-levelled his skills in order to support me in designing this book, and for his faith in each project that I birth.

In the Beginning, the Circle

In the beginning, the circle. One round opalescent sphere in the soft round depths of your mother's womb was fused with your father's seed, and life was born again in you.

Two tiny cells became four and then eight, until eventually you were a human body made up of billions. A constellation of life, beating to one heartbeat. Yours.

This was the first circle. You held in a bubble. Your body is still contained within its own bubble, your energy field. Your family are a larger circle that contains the bubble of you. Your community is another larger circle. All contained within the bubble of our earthly atmosphere. A blue green sphere spinning in space, orbited by a white moon, circling around a fiery spherical star.

Each has its own rhythms and cycles. Each one in constant motion. Just as your body has its own cycles of waking and sleeping, the in and out of your breath, the round of your menstrual cycle, the beating of your heart.

Now step back and see your whole lifetime before you. Each year a cycle, containing four seasons. Each season containing three months, each month itself a cycle of days. Each day has its own cycle, its own waxing and waning, its own rhythms of night and day. Each day marks a circle twice around the clock face. Each hour a cycle around the clock face, just as each minute is.

And now see all the circles connected with yours, each relationship you have, each project you start. Each is a world within a world. Each illness you experience, each stage of your life.

Welcome back to the wisdom of the circle.

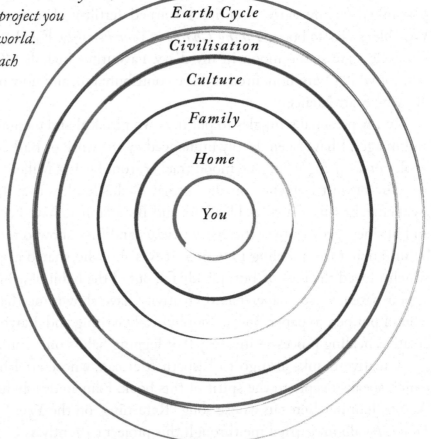

Earth Cycle

Civilisation

Culture

Family

Home

You

Full Circle Health
—
an introduction

For most of my adult life I have been trying to explore and express what it means to inhabit my cyclical female body.

I have picked up many tools and tried many approaches to charting my inner and outer life. I have charted my menstrual cycles, my moods, energy, habits, food intake, dreams... This was done in various written journals, sketchbooks, Excel spreadsheets, Life and Business Planners... not to mention my dream journal and cycle-tracking diary. So many books and scraps of paper piled beside my bed, with my computer balanced precariously on top. Keeping track of my health and life was almost a full-time job, but guaranteed I could never lay my hands on the right book at the right time.

I was filling in the first days of our Womancraft Publishing *Moon Dreams* charting diary, whilst simultaneously writing a book on women's health, when I realised that I needed an integrated space to reflect and capture every level of my body-mind. Something to stand testament to the feminine aspects of my body and inner life, which otherwise are hidden, silenced and untended. I needed a tool to help to retrain my body and mind, which would bring me into daily reconnection with them. I needed a system that would combine all these aspects into one easy-to-use format, so that I could have all that information in one place, at my fingertips. It needed to be something:

- That integrated all the parts of my health – cycle, physical, mental, energetic.

- That incorporated words and images.

- That was structured yet flexible, and allowed space for me to reflect on the fullness of my experience.

- That encouraged me to turn up to it daily.

- That enabled me to compile and easily track habits and symptoms in a monthly format, in order to get a detailed overview of my health.

What you are holding in your hands is the result.

Full Circle Health is an integration and expansion of all of my previous books and my own personal practice. It brings me full circle in my own work, combining my visual and written work, with my passion for women's health and empowerment. And it is a departure from my previous books, in that it offers an integral visual framework, and values images as much as words.

It is my deepest wish to help you celebrate your body and help you to reconnect with it. This book offers you hundreds of different ways in. All it takes is one to start you on your own path, or unblock the way.

I have a sense that this is your deepest wish too.

I'm curious. Why did you pick this book up? What called you to it? What silent wish did it answer? How can you get what you are yearning for from it?

I invite you to hold that intention as a silent prayer. To come back to it as your guiding light as you explore the material in this book. I am excited to see what happens when you commit a little time, every single day, to yourself. Watch what happens when you prioritise yourself in your life, when you consistently focus your awareness on your body and the world it inhabits.

For many of us our relationship with our bodies has been fraught. Often stemming from how we were taught to feel about them by those around us growing up. Our feelings about our health, about what it means to be sick, were shaped when we were young. Your symptoms may have been ignored and trivialised, or perhaps they were blown out of proportion and accompanied by hysterical, panicked parental reactions. Perhaps your life has been filled with operations, medication and medical interventions, or good health might have felt like your birthright. Perhaps your body felt like home until puberty hit, and from then on you have been fighting what feels like a losing battle against yourself. Perhaps you have just gotten the news that you are sick or pregnant, and are having to make major changes in your life.

One of this book's unique features is that it fits itself to your body, your needs. It meets you where you are.

I know I am not alone in often feeling a stranger in my own body and mind. For many of us our female bodies, our changing moods have been *terra incognita*. With no map and no compass, we have wandered lost.

No more.

You may have spent your life trying to understand how you work. I believe that the truth lies within you… nowhere else. But reading the book of your body, your mind, your moods and dreams can be challenging when you have not been taught how.

When you have not been taught to listen.

When you have not listened.

This journal is intended to help you to see, feel, value and record what your female life looks like.

We can see our bodies' outsides pretty easily, and as women have been taught to judge and value ourselves on their superficial appearance. With the rise of personal health devices so many metrics can be tracked for us – our heart rate, step count, body fat – but what of all the information that cannot be tracked digitally: our dreams, moods, the words that play on repeat in our heads, our menstrual phases, our energy – what of them?

My intention for this workbook is to share a practical tool that enables you to have information about your inner world at your fingertips – to become aware of the tides and cycles within you – and also of the wider cycles which impact your body, mind and soul. This book asks that you learn to listen to and honour the many different cycles of your life. It supports you in setting goals and healthy habits. It helps to make YOU the priority of your own life, which as busy women we can often struggle with, having been socialised to put everyone else's needs before our own. It holds space for your illness and suffering as well as your healing.

Full Circle Health is a creative way to journal each day, offering a framework to support you which is flexible enough to be tailored to your unique body, abilities, needs and cycles that you are experiencing right now. It offers a guided invitation and held space for you to show up, each day, to yourself, to your body. It encourages you to see and hear and touch the hundred different signals that you are receiving about the state of your health each day.

From experience I know that this gives you a sense of agency in your life, making you more aware of the multiple layers of you that exist. This is particularly important for those managing health issues where the body can all too quickly become medicalised, one-dimensional and its care commandeered by others. The *Full Circle Health* approach makes your healthcare and self-care central to your life, putting the observation of symptoms, as well as other aspects of your life, in your own hands.

Building embodied awareness requires the unlearning of many habits of a lifetime. Those of numbing ourselves, denying, negating or dramatising our physical and emotional feelings. At first this needs to be done explicitly and consciously, training our sensory awareness, heightening and learning to trust our intuitive insight, learning non-judgemental witnessing or awareness. This is what you will be doing as you chart daily. Key to your success is the act of noting down this information in an organised manner, rather than assuming you can and will remember it all. The act of writing (and drawing) this information is a journey of discovery in its own right. It is often in the process of putting pen to paper that realisations happen and connections between the internal and external become apparent to you.

Once this has become second nature, you can adapt the process to focus on emergent aspects of your life – such as a new way of eating or deepening your understanding of your unconscious self. It can support you with new health challenges as they arise and help you navigate new seasons of your female life such as new motherhood, menopause or coming back to your cycles after being on the pill.

Full Circle Health asks what happens when we pay attention to *all* the information that our bodies and minds are presenting us with? What happens when we dare to be truly present to the intricacies of our experiences? What happens when we integrate cyclical ways of knowing and being into our daily lives?

I am aware that each of us embarks upon this journey from a different starting point. We each arrive at this page with varying experiences of what it means to inhabit a woman's body and with different understandings of what it means to be a woman.

Most of us have been taught very little about what it means to live in a female body. The understanding is that we humans – men and women – are all pretty much the same.

The fixed, solid, permanent body and self are what we are taught to embody in our masculine defined culture. This seems to be easier for males whose bodies are less fluid and changeable. But for those of us in menstrual, childbearing bodies, trying to maintain this solidity in the midst of so much internal flux can be crazy making, and lead to ill health.

For women, reclaiming our own deep connection of circular energy and ways of being is crucial to our deeper understanding and acceptance of our bodies, our energy, our health and our consciousness. Our personal life cycles are embedded within the solar, lunar and earth-based life cycles. This book is a call to witnessing these cycles, connecting them, working with them on a deeper level than you have before. It is intended to work on two levels. Firstly as a mapping and reclamation of our physical women's bodies and their cycles of health. But also as a way to gain firsthand understanding of our consciousness, the deeper levels of being which we as women have more direct access to, through our cyclical bodies.

This book is an invitation to the wisdom of the circle. The circle is often considered a symbol for the constantly shifting energy of the feminine. In this book *feminine* refers to qualities which have often been ascribed to women, and have been sidelined in our culture: the wisdom of cycles, the feeling/emotional self, the unconscious, dreaming, creative self and the body.

In Western medicine specialist fields break the body into hundreds of discrete kingdoms, isolating the lungs from the guts, the eyes from the heart, as though they inhabited other sides of a planet, rather than shared the same fleshy home. As for dreams, feelings or the menstrual cycle, these are sidelined as irrelevant, rather than complex feedback loops between various levels of our being.

For true health and wellbeing we need to develop a lived, integrated, embodied awareness of our bodies' seasons. This book considers your health in a holistic manner, seeing all aspects of you as part of a whole, and seeing you as embedded in the world around you, rather than separate and autonomous, as we have been taught in our Western paradigm.

This book is held space for you to emerge in your fullness. It is a safe space for you to embody and express the whole of you. Inner and outer, healthy and ill. It is a women's circle, dedicated to you.

As women we have so few places that are devoted to our full emergence. I have made this book especially for women to see our bodies represented. It matters to have space that honours the cycles of womanhood. It matters to honour the emergent feminine in each of us.

Often our knowledge of ourselves is defined, and the parameters set, from the outside, using artificially calculated averages, or the male body as norm. You are not a norm. You are beautifully, individually you.

The norm co-opts our individuality, setting the benchmark for how we 'should' be. We come in all different body shapes and sizes, with differing configurations of organs, each with different levels of functioning. Our basal body temperature, our resting heart rate, our metabolism, our cycles (whether we have them and what length they are) all differ not only from person to person, but over the course of our lifetimes.

First and foremost this book is a way of establishing an intimate, integrated self-knowledge of your body – as it is NOW:

- ○ What normal feels like, looks like for YOU, at different times in your cycle, different times of year… It puts you back in touch with your body and allows you to learn and define your own baselines.

- ○ If you have a tendency to freak out at anything being wrong with your body, it gives you practice in simply observing without reacting.

- ○ It allows you to begin to recognise when something is building – perhaps it is persistent pain in one area, or a lack of energy – and to be able to respond to these subtler warnings before the problem develops further. Often we do not notice issues in our body until they have become big and hard to manage or requiring serious intervention. One of the aims of this health tracker is to get you more familiar with the subtler messages that your body provides that you may miss.

- ○ The real goal is to make building and maintaining health a habit in its own right – putting your health front and centre of your own life, rather than at the back of the queue.

Full Circle Health is big enough to take all of you. Don't hold back. Let these pages contain you so that they may help to reveal to you the wisdom of your body, the book of your own life.

It is time to listen to yourself deeply. To watch yourself like a lover. To step into the cycles of your life. To dedicate yourself fully to your body. To initiate yourself intimately into the experiment of your life.

What to Use this Book for

You may need to track your moods or mental health issues, or maybe it is your physical symptoms that are more pressing. You may be choosing to lose weight or strengthen your body after an injury. You may be breastfeeding, dealing with infertility or healing after a miscarriage. I have tried to suggest how this book may support a whole host of different women... and my dream is for you to find the way to use and personalise it in a way that supports YOU, your body, your health, your needs and your abilities best. For some, drawing and writing are healing and soothing, for others they are deeply stressful. For some, astrology is deeply meaningful, for others it has no place in their lives. Below I share just some of the ways you can use this book. I also share some sample pages so that you can see how several of these approaches would work in practice. But really the sky is the limit. I am fascinated to hear how you use this book. If you find ways to use it that I have not thought of please do share them with me, so that I can update future editions.

Chronic health issues – whether you are healing from cancer, living with CFS, ME, MS, diabetes, Lyme – there are so many aspects of your health you need to be aware of: energy levels, triggers, monitoring symptoms and medication as well as caring for your general health and fitness.

Diet – this may be losing weight, recovering from an eating disorder, an elimination diet, adapting to a new way of eating or tracking the impact of various foods such as caffeine, sugar, dairy or wheat on your body and energy levels.

Dream charting – you may be wanting to get into the habit of recording your dreams on waking, and explore how the moon's phase and your menstrual cycle affect your dreams. Or you may be struggling with trauma and needing to track nightmares.

Fertility/cycle awareness – this planner can be used to help you track your menstrual cycle, temperature, cervical fluid and feelings, along with the moon phases and libido to get a fuller picture of how your body changes throughout your cycle, finding your fertile window in which you want to conceive... or avoid conception.

Habit building – if you want to make it more likely that you will exercise every day, eat to support your health, do rehabilitation exercises or mindfulness practice, logging your behaviours, setting goals and reviewing your progress is a vital way to make yourself accountable as you build new behaviours into your daily life.

Managing mental health issues – your mood, energy levels, physical health, stressors, anniversaries and times of year, menstrual cycle and even the moon can impact your mental health. When you track your shifting moods and energy levels over the course of the day, week and year you can pick up on danger signals which warn of relapse. You begin to observe the impact of your sleep, self-care practices and exercise on your mental health, helping you to turn around negative spirals more quickly and knowing when to call in support. This planner is a great way of collecting and sharing information with health professionals, giving easy-to-access, accurate records of symptoms, their frequency and severity.

Medication tracking – keep note of which drugs you are taking, what amount, and side effects you are experiencing. This is especially important when increasing or decreasing dosage or adding or removing a medication from your current regime.

Post-partum – whether you are wanting to log your baby's sleeping, feeding and waking patterns so that you can also schedule your own rest and self-care. Or perhaps you're weaning, wanting to lose some baby weight or to build more exercise and outdoor time into your life. Like many new mums often your own health and recovery from birth gets put at the bottom of the priority list. Charting these will help you to focus every day on your own body.

Pregnancy – note how many weeks gestation you are, your symptoms of the day such as Braxton Hicks or spotting, your baby's position, engagement of the head, or any issues you want to raise with your doctor or midwife. Note down dreams of the birth or baby.

Self-care tracking – often we can treat self-care (exercise, eating well, taking a bath, creative time, time for prayer and reflection...) as a bonus, an optional extra when everything on our to-do list is done. This planner asks what happens when you prioritise it and build it into your daily schedule.

Sleep tracking – for those who struggle to get enough sleep, or who have problems getting to or staying asleep, charting allows you to note the number of wakings, medication, your wake and sleep times, and how food, exercise or other habits may be impacting the quality of your sleep.

Spiritual health – chart your menstrual cycle, moon phase, chakras, intuitive hits. Note the main astrological phenomena and fill in the key phrases from today's horoscope. Pull a tarot card or affirmation and write it in one of the large circles and create a daily mandala in the other, add in your archetype and word of the day, chart whether you have done your yoga or meditation practice for the day, and of course log your dreams.

Stress tracking – if stress is impacting your health negatively, this is a great way to note stresses as they happen and how your body responds.

How to Use the Book — getting started

Full Circle Health revolves around two basic practices: your Daily Charting Pages and your Monthly Review Pages. Each day you will take stock of where you are physically, mentally, emotionally and spiritually using the 35 blank charting and journaling pages laid out for you later on. To tie all of this precious information together, there then follows a set of simple exercises in the Monthly Review Pages. (You are free to photocopy these blank pages for your own personal use, purchase a printable pdf version at shop.womancraftpublishing.com, or if you prefer to have them all together in one beautiful bound volume, the *Full Circle Health: 3-Month Charting Journal* is also available from your favourite retailer: ISBN 978-1-910559-383).

The main instruction I have for you is to use this book is in a spirit of curiosity and exploration, openness to discovery, free from shame or self-judgement. You are invited to spill yourself onto the page – in all your messiness, your contradictions, your uncertainty and imperfection. It's okay to make mistakes, the more the better. It's okay to erase, scribble out, start again tomorrow, try something new, change your focus half way through the month. You need to figure it out as you go along. All the guidance I am giving you here is to share my vision as to how it can be used, so that you have the courage to start. After that it's all yours. There is no wrong way. Except to not use it at all.

This book is supposed to reflect you. I have allowed as much flexibility as I can, whilst including as many of us as possible. You may have one leg or no breasts, you may be heavier or slimmer than the image shown, you may not have cycles... Where you differ, be sure to honour yourself, adapt this image to make it your own so that you see yourself reflected fully within it, so that what is generic does not feel like a judgement on you.

I felt it important not to impose a start date on you. It takes 28 days to make a new habit, so it is intended that you chart daily for a month. You may choose to do a calendar month, a lunar month or if you are menstruating or on the pill, the duration of one cycle. A full month is a great way to get into the habit of checking in with your body.

I recommend working in pencil. And so you don't worry about making mistakes – get an eraser too! Coloured pencils will not go through the paper, you can build them up and blend them and they will not blot or spread. If you do want to use a pen, then ballpoints and biros tend to work better on this paper than fibre tips which may show through the page.

I have always used images in my own personal healing work, but my professional work was divided between my writing and my image work. It was only when I was compiling and teaching my most recent e-course, *WORD+image*, that I realise just how important it is, in healing, in wholing that we use words and images together as a way of tapping into our full awareness. Please do take the opportunity to personalise your pages – doodle, draw, colour – make them your own, make them beautiful, make them messy. Please don't be precious with this book – let your words and images reflect your mood and what is happening in your life now. If you cannot find words for what you are feeling, try images. They don't need to make any logical sense. They don't have to be perfect... or even good, but the simple act of trying to translate your feelings into something visible, holds immense power.

As a side note, notice when you feel drawn to use colour and when black and white is what feels safest or most appropriate. Notice when you only use words, and when images or symbols emerge for you.

Energy

Often in this book I refer to 'energy'. When I do, I mean primarily your felt sense of your own life-force. When it is depleted we feel tired, when it is full we feel we can take on the world. Our energy is impacted primarily by:

- Our sleep – both duration and quality.
- The physical fuel that creates it – what we eat and drink.
- Our activities and experiences.
- Our health – illness usually drains our life-force.
- The environment around us.

If you find yourself getting stuck when thinking about your energy, ask yourself:

- What gives me energy?
- What drains me?
- How do I recharge?
- How often do I need to recharge?
- How do I spend my energy on an average day?

This is a great starting point in getting to know your body better.

Sickness often happens when our energy is depleted – through eating poorly, physical or mental exhaustion, overwork or an overtaxed immune system. One of the things you will be doing as you chart your health is monitoring your energy levels.

Cycles

Energy is always moving and changing form. This can be chaotic, but in most life-forms it is regulated into a particular dynamic flow. Most energetic processes tend to move in cycles of expansion and contraction.

Our bodies are in constant, rhythmic change. But because so much of this is happening beneath our waking consciousness we can often feel overwhelmed and confused by the seeming turbulence of our bodies and unpredictability of our moods. However, when we begin to notice the pattern of these cycles, their repetitive nature, their connection to nature beyond us, we can begin to feel not victims unprepared for the weather, but like adventurers of days gone by, who navigate by nature – the pull of the tides, the placing of the stars and the gathering storm clouds.

In this book you can choose to monitor several bio-energetic processes, perhaps your blood sugar if you are diabetic, your mood if you have mental health issues, energy levels if you have a chronic health issue, your menstrual cycle, your wake-sleep cycle… Take a few moments to think over the key energy cycles which currently get out of balance and negatively impact your life – fill them in here:

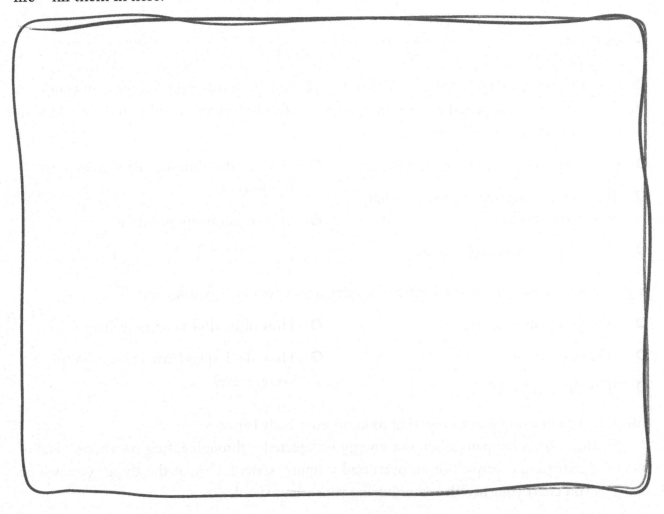

And which natural cycles are you particularly sensitive to? The weather, the moon, the movements of the planets, pollen, temperature, humidity?

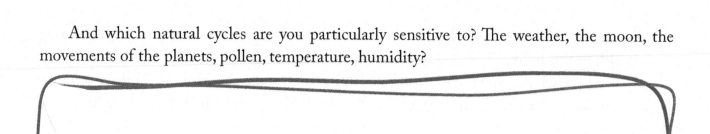

And now think about the cycles of time. Which times of year seem to have a cyclical impact on you? Which times of the month, or the day are significant for you? They might be anniversaries of birth or death, end of the month when money is tight, your pre-menstrual time, times when your partner is away, the bedtime routine. Note them down here:

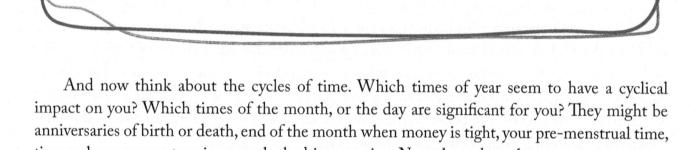

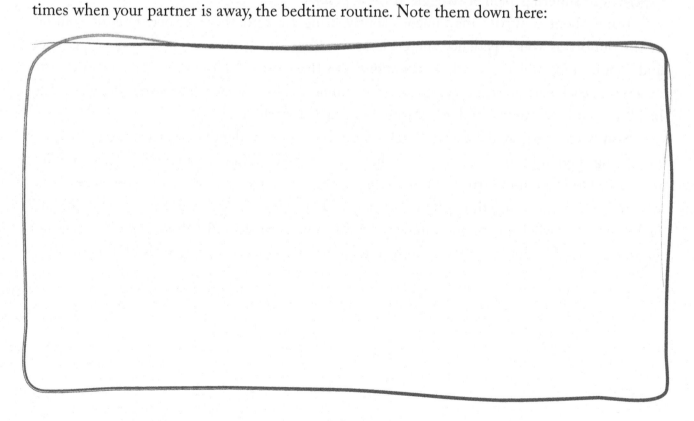

Becoming aware of these helps you to decide what you will focus on as you begin charting your health in this book.

As you log each day, and then transfer this information onto the Monthly Tracker you may begin to notice patterns and interconnections that are harder to see when you are just living the details of daily life.

Cycle Circles

On the facing page are some of the cycles that many of us experience. Take a moment to mentally and energetically travel through each Cycle Circle. Reflect on how you tend to feel and respond to the aspects of each. You may want to write in some of the key feelings and associations that emerge for each one. Perhaps colour each stage in a colour that you connect with it. There are a couple of blank circles overleaf you can fill in if there are key cycles of yours that are not shown here.

Once you have done this with each of the Cycle Circles, consider which part of each of the cycles is your favourite? And which do you struggle with most? The places you most enjoy could be thought of as your Comfort Zones. These are perhaps what you have been taught by your family or culture are the most desirable. They might also be those that your body/mind find easiest and most pleasurable. Reflect on how you feel during these. And then reflect on the Discomfort Zones. Have you been taught that they are undesirable? How has your body/mind experienced suffering, pain or struggle at these points?

Think about how you may unconsciously bring forward these associations of comfort or discomfort as you experience the cycle again. How much does your previous experience and conditioning impact your later experiences of these cycles? How can you free yourself to experience each part of each cycle as it is, in its fullness? How can you allow your body/mind to be immersed more fully in and learn from each stage of each cycle?

Now look again at the Cycle Circles. See the correspondences between them, imagine overlaying them on top of each other so that each of the quadrants is aligned. Take some time to reflect. Do you tend to struggle most often in the first stage of a cycle? Or are you someone who resists or tries to rush through the last stage? Do you lose direction and focus in the middle, or become overwhelmed by the intensity of full moon/ovulation/birth stage? How can you support yourself in finding greater comfort, focus or ease in your current areas of discomfort?

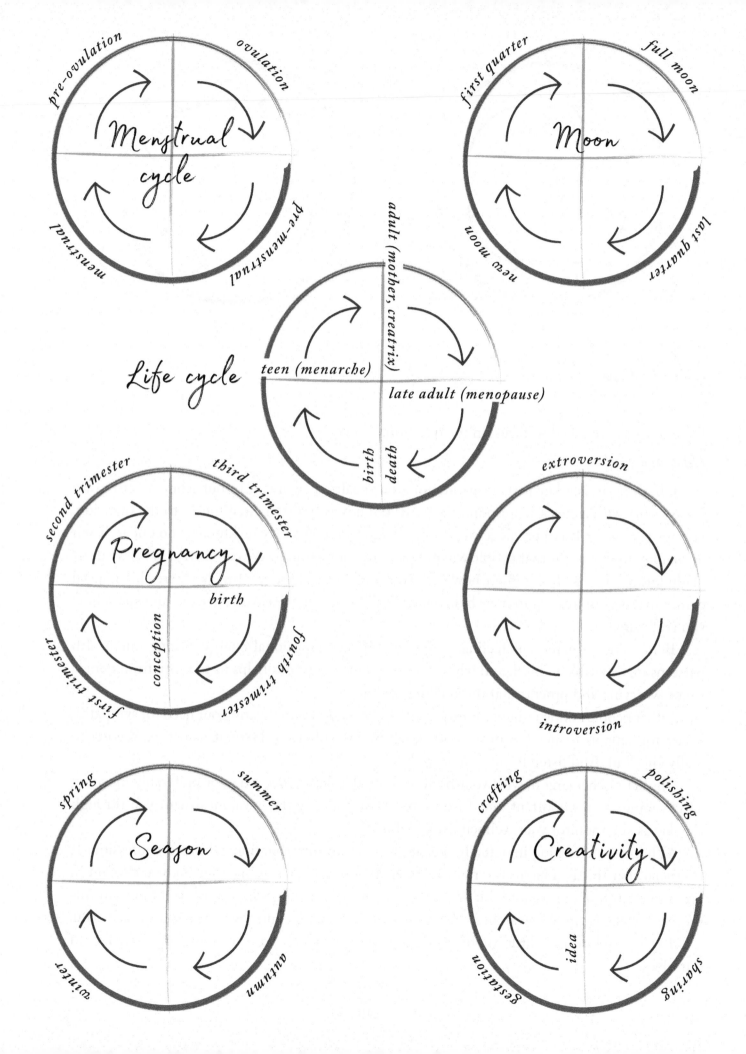

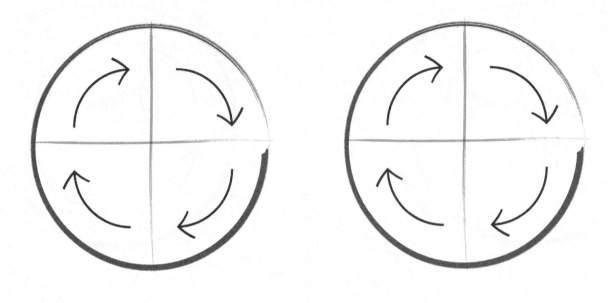

Checking In

Each day you are asked to focus on the question:

How are you?

Checking in is a key part of maintaining our health as women. In our women's group we always start with a check in, responding freely and honestly, often circuitously, to the question: *how are you really?* It is a privilege we as women rarely get. We may feel there is no one to listen or that no one cares. Or that people will judge us for complaining. We can worry that if we don't really know what is wrong, then how can we begin to verbalise it? This is where this journal comes in. You can turn up to it each day, and it will bear witness as you check in and share how you really are.

Being able to name our feelings helps to shift our emotional energy. Seeing our health patterns made visible in black and white over the course of weeks helps us to move from denial, vague worrying and procrastination to taking action.

Other people asking us how we are can add layers of drama, activating our need for sympathy, desire for support or need to prove how much we are suffering. Here, it is just us. We get to really check in. And listen to the responses.

The act of checking in with your body and mind at least once a day, or preferably morning and evening, is an important one. In time you learn to carry this awareness with you through the day as you monitor your wellbeing and habits.

What does 'checking in' actually mean? It is not an interrogation or forced confession. It is crucial that this is done in the right manner. You are not observing your body and mind in order to control, shame or criticise them. Rather you are learning who you are right now, in this moment, by being in full awareness of your body, mind, energy and the world as it impacts you.

Let us explore in a little more depth the ways in which we can know and understand ourselves:

- The logical mind, located in the brain, which is so exalted and cultivated and dominant in our culture: analytical, deductive, but devoid of feeling and emotion. This tends to be black and white, it likes to use labels, to diagnose, to apply systems and frameworks. It is extremely useful, but needs to be used in balance with other ways of knowing.

- The nervous system, connected to the spine and a network of millions of nerves gives us immediate sensory feedback in terms of pain or pleasure.

- The feeling self, usually experienced in the belly/solar plexus region. This is our instinctual 'gut feeling'. We have to feel it physically and then translate that information into words or images. This pre-verbal, animal self can easily be shut down or overruled by the logical mind.

- The electromagnetic energy field around us that can be disturbed by influences both inner and outer, this is not felt directly with the body, nor known with the mind, and yet we have an awareness of it, some of us more than others.

- The witness self which enables us to step beyond our immediate thoughts and feelings and see ourselves with detachment – often with greater wisdom and compassion and insight. But this disembodied manner of being can mean that we become disengaged from our physical bodies and feelings. This spiritual sense can be a great gift, but also a means of escaping from the physical world, of keeping ourselves safe and detached from our reality.

As you check in and reflect on your body, mind and energy, be sure that you find ways of moving between these different ways of knowing. Each has powerful and important insight.

This book is based on meeting yourself where you are. Getting to know the ebbs and flows of your energy and health – physical, mental, emotional – and understanding yourself as a dynamic, complex, ever-changing being. We do this by learning to regularly check in.

Checking in and charting what you discover is a two-way process. You are not just acting as a detached, objective witness. You are deeply invested in what you are studying: it is your body and your life. Everything that you observe responds to the act of being watched. Patterns emerge. You see more deeply and clearly than before. Your feminine self learns that she will be listened to, respected, trusted, honoured. Her messages and wisdom are being heeded, perhaps for the first time. She responds to this and blooms. A state of equilibrium and flow becomes established as your default setting, where once there was internal discord or stagnation. You begin to see how you can move through blockages, discard unsupportive habits and inhabit your body/mind more fully.

Wherever you are, let's start from there. I want to support you in developing self-awareness and enable you to meet your body and energy where they are, as you learn to observe yourself as a compassionate, caring ally. Prepare for self-knowledge. Open to miracles. Allow for healing.

How to Use the Daily Charting Pages

Perhaps you have an idea of what you are wanting to track and how. But if you are feeling a little stuck, if you're looking at all the empty circles on the blank Daily Charting Pages later on wondering what to put in them, how to use them... this section will help you figure it out.

I need to stress again that there is no *correct* way. There is also no obligation to fill in every space. The Circles and Grid are there as a framework to support your charting, your process and your health. Each of our needs are different. Your needs, focus and desires will probably change over the course of your charting journey. Some days you will have more time, energy or desire to chart than others, some days will be more eventful than others.

Let's take a look at a Daily Charting Page. You will see it is broken down into various sections that we will go through step by step.

Starting from the top you have:

O **Moons:** four medium and two slightly smaller circles.

O **Buttons:** two sets of four small circles on each side of the page.

O **Body Maps:** front and back views of a female body.

O **Gauges:** two semi-circles.

O **Mirrors:** two large circles.

O **Lines:** on the outside of the two Mirrors.

O **Timepiece:** the hourglass shape between the two Mirrors.

O **Daily Grid:** at the bottom of the page.

Throughout the book each of these aspects will be capitalised so that you know when they are referring to particular parts of the chart. The rest of this chapter will take you through how you might use each of them.

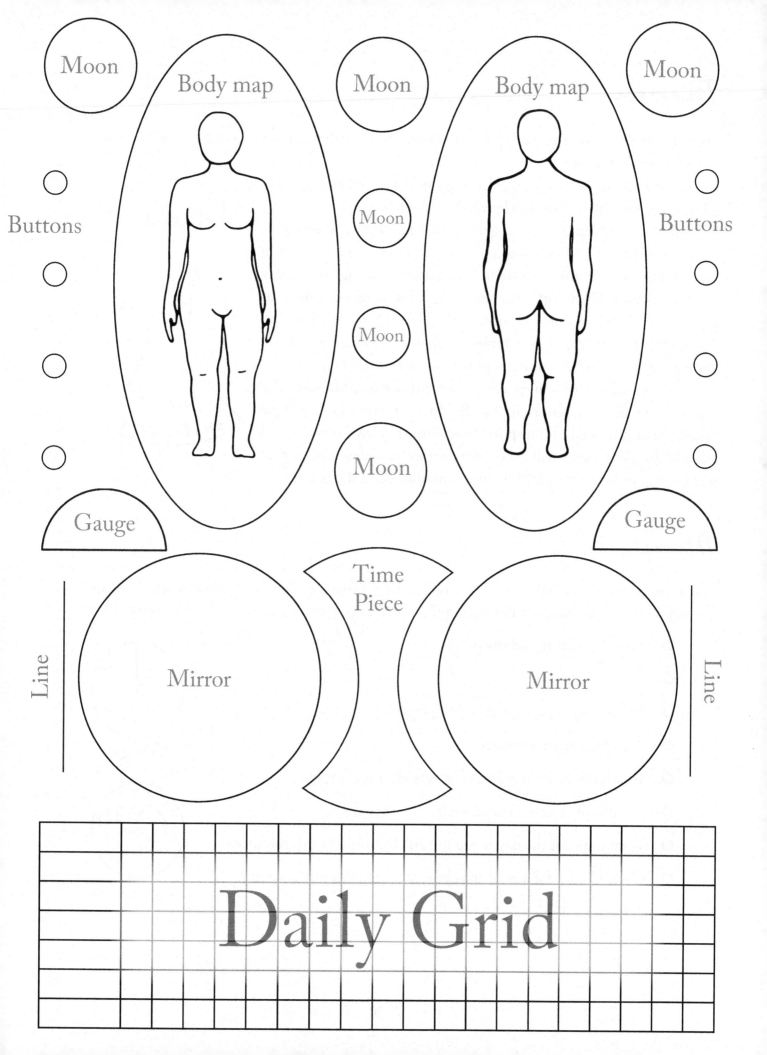

Moon

Body map

Moon

Moon

Body map

Moon

Buttons

Moon

Buttons

Moon

Gauge

Gauge

Time
Piece

Line

Mirror

Mirror

Line

Daily Grid

Timepiece

I recommend that you start each page by adding the day's date. I tend to add it to the Timepiece in the centre of the page.

Whilst just about everything else is optional, the ability to quickly reference a page by its date will be really valuable for you.

I feel it is helpful to have a general outline of what this day is, before we check in to see how our body is responding to it. You may choose to add any important information relating to the day – anniversaries, big events, the weather, season, moon phase or astrological events of note, the time you woke... You can either do this in the Timepiece, or preferably in separate Moons so that the Timepiece does not become overcrowded or overwhelming.

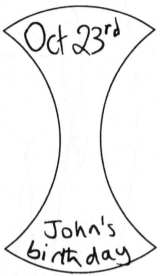

I use a Northern Hemisphere perspective when addressing the seasons and months, sisters in the Southern Hemisphere will be familiar with the need to transpose these onto your own seasons, and tropical dwelling sisters will have their own wet and dry seasons that will correspond with the shifting cycles mentioned in the book.

Moons

There are two sizes of Moon – four large and two smaller. Obviously choose which to use depending on the amount of information they need to contain. With the Moons you might log:

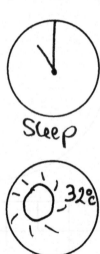

- Time of waking and sleeping.
- The moon phase.
- The season, weather and/or temperature.
- Astrological information.
- Your level of introversion/extroversion using a spiral.
- The day of your menstrual cycle.
- Total steps for the day if you use an electronic health monitor.
- Cycle Circles for any of the cycles you are currently tracking.

You may choose to use the left hand side of the page for the morning and the right for the evening. So taking the example of the weather you may choose to:

- Draw in symbols like those you see in newspaper or television weather reports using a sun, clouds, snow...

- Write down the weather, e.g. 'windy', 'blizzard'.

- Note the temperature or humidity.

- Note the pollen count or air pollution.

With the moon you can:

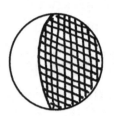

- Draw in the moon's phase.

- Note whether it is waxing or waning.

- Note which astrological sign it is in.

- Note if it is a super moon, eclipse, blue moon or other lunar event.

For the seasons you can either:

- Write in the season, and any notable festival such as Summer Solstice or Christmas.

- Draw in a wheel of the year. Subdivide the year into 12 months, like a clock face, where midsummer is at 12 o'clock and midwinter at 6 o'clock and mark where you are using a clock hand.

The action of filling out the moon phase, weather and season each day seeks to ground you firmly in the physical reality that your body inhabits. In a culture dominated by indoor spaces and screens, and especially for those who live in cities and towns whose days are more influenced by the traffic than the moon phase, it can be easy to ignore or minimise these factors. But the weather has a big impact on our moods. We find ourselves feeling very different on a hot day to a mild one. The difference between a hurricane or a day of incessant drizzle still impacts our day's plans, stress levels and health in myriad ways. As we begin to pay more attention to these natural phenomena we begin to see just how much they shift and change, how our 'internal weather' and health often reflect the outer weather.

As we begin to contextualise our health and inner cycles within the bigger picture of larger natural cycles, we start making connections between what might seem like disconnected factors, so that we are empowered to solve our own puzzles and embrace our own unique health issues.

The Body Scan

After filling in the day's external factors, I recommend that you continue each charting session with a Body Scan. This may take just a few seconds to scan quickly over your body to get a sense of any areas of tension or discomfort. Or you may choose to do a detailed Body Scan meditation.

The Body Scan is a meditative technique in its own right and helps to centre and root our energy into our physical bodies. For those of us who struggle with anxiety, dissociation or dysmorphia this is a really important way of starting the day, helping us to feel as safe as we can being here in our physical bodies.

The Body Scan will help you to see what areas you are ignoring, suppressing or unaware of in the course of your daily life: where, what and why are you not allowing yourself to feel.

How to do the Body Scan

I suggest that you start at the top of your head, as most of us usually spend our time trapped in our heads. Our heads are also the source of a huge amount of our sensory feedback and it is often easiest to start by putting our awareness here.

In the Body Scan we are looking for both physical and energetic symptoms. Be sure with each body part that you move through the various levels of being: skin, nerves, muscle, bones, organs, and your inner energy and then back out of your body to your energy field. You may choose to do this with each part, or check in with your whole body on the skin level, then the muscle level and so forth, moving inwards. This is all about learning to pick up on the information or signals that your body sends you: pain, numbness, heat, cold, swelling, tingling, words, images and associations. We are learning to read the body and gain information and insight from our bio-energetic beings.

We have been educated to break our body into distinct parts, like the parts of a car. But the truth of the human body is far, far more complex, with many parts interacting or with interconnected functioning. So be aware of this as you scan. Pay attention to the joints and internal passages that have little solidity, but ensure the flow of energy, food, fluids and sensation around your body:

- Sinuses
- Digestive tract
- Airways
- Vagina and womb
- Lymph drainage
- Blood vessels

Ways of Knowing

Take notice of your default way of knowing/experiencing your body. For example, when Body Scanning do you close your eyes or keep them open? If you close your eyes, do you notice them moving as though looking at the different parts of your body – so when you are examining your left side, they are looking left?

Read through the various 'ways of knowing' below and reflect on them. Can you and do you switch easily between these ways of knowing your body? Which do you trust, and which don't you trust? Do you combine aspects of them? If not, challenge yourself to try doing it a different way and see what emerges for you. Ways of knowing include:

- Technological testing – such as blood tests, taking a temperature, using apparatus to test the body.

- Logical mind – putting together symptoms into a coherent pattern to explain an ailment.

- Visual – looking at your body in the mirror.

- Physical touch – like the way we check for broken bones or breast lumps, physically palpating the body with our fingers.

- Disembodied witness – do you imagine yourself standing outside of your body and seeing your body as though it were in the mirror? Or do you float above or behind your body from a disembodied perspective and see things intuitively. This incorporates our spiritual and creative powers.

- Inner-visual – 'seeing' your body in your mind's eye. It is likely that colours or images come up for you. You may be able to visualise each organ and your internal structures and 'see' what state of health they are in.

- Inner-feeling – do you feel your body from the inside, staying totally rooted in it, getting your information from felt sensation only?

Each perspective gives you information in different ways. When we feel our bodies with our fingers the information we receive: hard, soft, lumpy, rough… is different from when we intuitively witness our bodies and sense colours, images or words. Can you connect the wisdom of each of these ways of knowing your body to get a fuller picture of your embodied self?

In this way you may be able to watch, in real time, the beginnings of a migraine or a downwards mood spiral, the onset of an infection, the growth of a lump, how anxiety is presenting in your body physically, the healing of an injury…

A note is needed here: for those of us who struggle with panic, health anxiety and with tendencies towards hypochondria, remember that we are simply bringing our awareness to our bodies, without fear, without the need to respond immediately or worry about every ache and pain. There is no need to rush to the doctors, unless you feel you are in immediate danger.

The intention behind the Body Scan is about building awareness of your physical and energetic body, to build a feeling of comfort, ease and familiarity with each part of your body, and it as a whole. This enables you to observe as things morph and change, to see the patterns that may emerge within the menstrual cycle or the solar cycle. First observe, with openness and curiosity, gather your information. For those who find attending a health professional stressful, this is a good way of information gathering in advance of taking the plunge and making an appointment.

Once you have scanned your body, next you need to make a note of what you have found. You do this on the Body Map.

Body Mapping

At the heart of *Full Circle Health* is the Body Map. For many of us even this – identifying yourself with this physical image – is powerful work: a visual reminder that you inhabit a physical form.

The back and front views of the body are shown so that you have a 360 degree vision of yourself. Sidedness does matter. Firstly because the physical location of pain is obviously crucial when discussing issues with doctors. But furthermore, your dominant hand will impact how you use the whole of your body, and is the side that is under more physical pressure, as well as being stronger. The sides of the brain are, just to remind you, crossed over – so the left is the logical rational brain (in very general terms) responsible for language and controlling the right side of the body, it is associated with the masculine. The right brain is the 'creative', image-based brain and is connected to the left side of the body and is associated with the feminine.

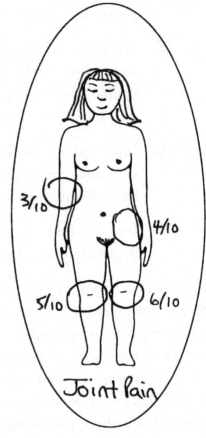

When filling in your Body Map you might want to create your own 'Charting Key' of different symbols and colours (see later section) so that you can refer back to it and ensure consistency between days. So, for example, you may choose to use pink for painful places, red for heat and blue for cold. You might want to use symbols for what the pain feels like, arrows for the direction it is moving in.

O   You may decide to log all your physical symptoms on one of the figures and the energetic on the other.

O   You can colour in the places that are feeling sore, tired or sensitive on the body diagram, using words outside the body – but within the oval shape – to describe these symptoms.

O   You might want a different focus each day – so one day you just map your skin, the next your muscles, the next your bones and joints, the next your energy.

- You might choose to do a temperature map like those you see in thermal images, from blue for the coldest areas, through green, yellow, orange and red.

- You may choose to use one for your morning check in and one for an evening check in.

Gauges

Once you have done the Body Scan and Map you are more attuned with how you are feeling and what your energy levels are like.

Fill in the Gauge for how energetic you feel right now. You'll note that it's marked like a fuel gauge in a vehicle – are you full, half full or getting close to empty? You may choose to use the Gauge with a red/amber/green traffic light system or rank your energy levels from 1-5 or use a Moon and fill it according to energy levels. Charting our energy is particularly important for those with autoimmune illnesses, who are pregnant, new mothers and women in the last part of the menstrual cycle. You can use one for the morning and evening. Obviously your energy fluctuates throughout the day, but if you have a regular check in time each day, this will be a reliable indicator. If you wish to chart your energy levels continuously throughout the day I suggest you use the Daily Grid.

Mirrors

The intention for these larger circles is to act as windows or mirrors onto areas of your life that need your focus, or that you need to see reflected back to you. They can be used as:

- Spotlight – you may choose to focus on one part of your body that there isn't enough detail on the Body Map for. So, for example if you are struggling with your hands or feet, or an internal organ you may choose to sketch it here and do the Body Mapping exercise focused on the intricacies of this part of your body.

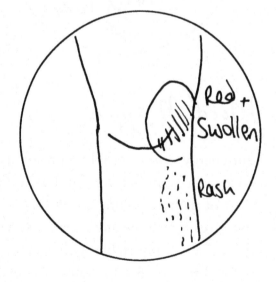

- Headspace – show, using words or images, what is going on in your head. You might choose to note down key words, feelings or themes that are dominating your day, do a mind map, draw a picture of your brain with all the things you are thinking about, the day's major events or stressors...

- Note to Self – this might be reminders for how to treat a medical condition, key words or phrases that have come up for you today, your horoscope, a tarot card you have drawn, your daily gratitudes...

- Pie Chart – you can use these to log any pie chart your brilliant mind comes up with!

- Feelings Wheel (see below).

- Doodle – use it as a space to create a daily doodle, zentangle or mandala. This is a great way of centring yourself and seeing what images are wanting to emerge from your subconscious.

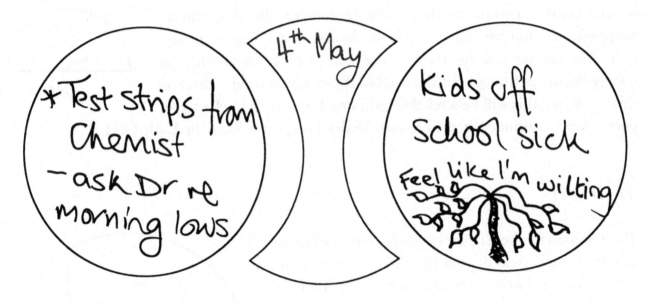

Mood Mapping

Our energy is most visibly expressed through our moods, which can be quite changeable. Our moods can be important pointers to the current state of our underlying mental health issues. Most of us have feeling states that we find hard to accept or articulate. The Feelings Wheel tool gives us a non-judgemental way of becoming aware of all our feelings, not just those that we are comfortable with. Some of us have emotions that can become excessive, which we need to monitor, for some it is mania, for others anger or anxiety. When we see that one feeling is predominating for several days, or even is off the scale, we need to take action and seek professional help. For those who struggle with alexithymia (a difficulty with being able to read emotions in ourselves or others), are on the autistic spectrum or those who struggle with interpreting mixed-feeling states, the tools you are learning here can be an invaluable way of identifying how you are feeling, in all its complexity.

You may choose to do a Feelings Wheel in the morning and evening, or when you are in a flurry of heightened emotion or agitation and needing to get a sense of what is going on. Kind of like a pie chart, you can use it for logging all the different feelings and intensity you are experiencing. You may use it to help you to move through a challenging time in your life such as a period of depression or grief, acting as a reflection of your inner state, so that you can see yourself improve over time.

To make a Feelings Wheel, divide one of the Mirrors into quarters, and then into eighths. Then draw two concentric circles inside, so it is divided into three sizes of circle. The inner ring is low intensity, the outer rim is maximum intensity. Then along each of the lines, write a different feeling. Then do a small cross on each line to correspond to how you are feeling, then join these up to make a sort of spider's web. Or you can shade in each segment to the required level, as you see below.

Feelings you may want to chart include:

O Angry

O Sad/grief

O Happy/joyful

O Excited/manic

O Anxious/fearful

O Depressed/numb/bored

O Peaceful/relaxed/calm

O Paranoid

O Overwhelmed

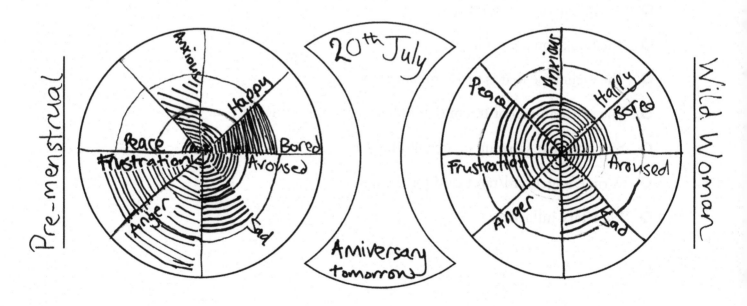

27

A growing awareness of your emotional energy and mood allows you to say that you are feeling angry, rather than enact your anger on someone; to express your feeling of anxiety rather than shutting down. Expression can be verbal, written, drawn, or kinaesthetic dependent on your mood. The explosive energy of anger usually needs a fast, loud, explosive outlet such as banging, hitting, stamping, whereas the erratic, swirling energy of anxiety usually needs holding, stroking, calming, a sense of safe containment. Once we know this and can recognise it, we can care for ourselves more quickly, and these energies can be far less damaging, both to ourselves and those around us. Furthermore, we begin to see the connections between the inner and outer worlds, how we take on energies from others. We also begin to see how what is in our headspace can become physical symptoms.

But perhaps the best reason for doing a Feelings Wheel is to bear witness to the fact that our energies and feelings do shift from day to day and moment to moment, though they can feel overwhelming and eternal at the time.

Lines

You may choose to use the two lines on either side of the Mirrors to record what is influencing you most. This may be:

- Your word of the day – it may be something that jumps out at you whilst you are reading, or when someone is speaking to you. What word holds strong energy for you today?

- An affirmation or mantra.

- The book you are reading.

- The archetype that is predominant for you.

- The spirit animal or totem that holds strong medicine for you.

- Symbols that show up or are guiding you.

- A rune/angel card/tarot card for the day.

- Planetary influences.

Buttons

These smaller circles are intended to act as a checklist for something you are tracking over the course of the month. They are preferably something that you do – or aim to have done – once a day. If you want to log something several times in a day or track it in more detail, I recommend using the Daily Grid area, which we will come to next.

You will need to write what each is beside or below each Button. Then you can tick (check), cross or colour in each. The Buttons I use are:

O Play
O Pray
O Create
O Sex (yes)

O Exercise
O Chocolate (yes, really!)
O Read
O Vitamins

☑ Create   O Sex

O Play   O Chocolate

O Meditate   O Yoga

☑ Walk   ☑ Check in with Friends

These are all things I need to do regularly to stay happy, healthy and in balance. When I am regularly missing the majority of these from my life I start to get stressed, depressed, blocked and shut down. The act of missing these practices says that my focus is not on my health and wellness, it has gone elsewhere – either because I am too busy, or because my mental health is slipping. Too much of any of them might mean I am using one as a coping mechanism which also pushes me out of balance. Others might include:

O Medication
O Meditation

O Stretch
O Gratitude

O Nap
O Run

You may also choose to use the Buttons to track symptoms that recur frequently and need close monitoring, or medications you need to take. So, for example if you are suffering from an autoimmune condition your list might look something like this:

O Headache
O Tired
O Glands up

O Temperature
O Aching muscles
O Brain fog

O Tremors

And you check off each symptom that you experience over the course of the day.

Daily Grid

The first longer box is for you to write down the category you are tracking – for example 'Energy' or 'Screen time'. Each smaller box represents an hour. Mark down the hours based on what hours you live by: I know some who rise at 4 and others at 11, so make it fit *your* day. You can write the numbers above each of the vertical grid lines. The Daily Grid allows space for a 19 hour day – if your days are longer than this, you may want to look at seeing how you can get some more sleep! There are many ways to fill in your Daily Grid including:

- Using symbols, initials, ticks, stars or coloured stickers.

- Writing in data – miles walked, steps taken, blood sugar levels, pollen counts...

- Shading in boxes for activities lasting half an hour or more.

- Using the row as a line chart to log fluctuating energy or pain levels.

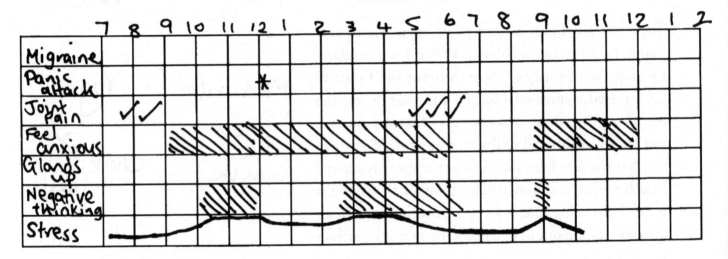

Charting Key

I strongly advise building a Charting Key for yourself, like the sort you would see in the corner of a map. You will find your Charting Key sheet before the blank Daily Charting Pages. A key provides a reference point for the symbols and shorthand most frequently used in order to quickly read and understand your charts. It also helps you to fill in information consistently, in a time and space efficient manner. Your key may include:

- Colour coding
- Symbols
- Emojis

- Ticks, crosses, asterisks
- Initials or abbreviations

Make it your own, make it fun and easy to use and reference.

On my Daily Grid I have developed certain codes to break down information into more detailed data. So, for example, in my water-intake column I have different beverages to see if I am overdoing it on sugar or caffeine any day:

T – tea   W – water

C – coffee   J – juice

For my screen time I have subdivided it so I can see clearly and quickly where I have spent my time. This matters to me, because using my phone and computer in the evening are liable to adversely impact my ability to fall asleep and the quality of my dreams, whereas the TV doesn't seem to. Too much computer work during the day tends to drain my energy and leave me feeling lethargic. Sometimes screen time is used as self-care, such as going to the movies with friends. Whereas at other times, like watching mindless TV when I'm sick, it is a way of avoiding being present and dealing with what is wrong.

So my screen time Grid row is shaded to cover all screen time, with each type of screen time noted.

TV – television   C – computer   P – phone

You could also choose to use a different colour for each.

Now you understand what each of the parts of the Daily Charting Pages can be used for, let's take a look at some examples, along with a brief explanation of each.

Charting Key

▢	1 portion of wheat	TV	Television
⊌	1 glass of water	P	Phone
✳	Low stress	C	Computer
✳✳	Medium Stress	ⓒ	Anxiety
✳✳✳	High Stress		

Sample Charting Pages

Sample Chart 1 — Charting the Menstrual Cycle

This woman has chosen to log her wake and sleep times on the top row of Moons. The central Moons log the moon phase, days of her menstrual cycle, the phases of menstrual cycle and where she is on them. Her introversion spiral shows she is feeling introverted but moving out towards the world. The Lines show the menstrual phase she is in and the related archetype.

On the left she is using the Buttons to track her goals and on the right, her symptoms.

She has used the Gauges to log her energy levels at 9am and 7pm. She has used the Mirrors to create Feelings Wheels at the same times.

In the Daily Grid she has tracked her energy over the course of the day, stress, water, self-care, screen time, as well as her temperature and cervical fluid for fertility charting.

Sample Chart 2 — Charting Pregnancy

This woman tracks pollen as she has hayfever and asthma. She also tracks the moon and weather. It's hard being hot when you're heavily pregnant!

In the middle Moons she tracks her weight, the engagement of the baby's head, and how many weeks and days pregnant she is. She uses the Buttons to track her self-care and the Gauges to track her morning and evening energy.

The Mirrors show her baby's position, and the affirmation she is using today.

She is using the Daily Grid to track the Braxton Hicks contractions and baby's kicks, as well as her naps and exercise.

Sample Chart 3 — Charting Post-Partum

This busy mama does not have much time on her hands, but she is using the Daily Charts to set reminders to herself of self-care activities she can do. You can see from the Body Map she's feeling low and has mastitis, so has used one of the Mirrors to note down the treatment advice her midwife gave her.

In the Daily Grid she is logging her baby's feeds and napping when he is. She is keeping a careful eye on her pain levels, hydration and temperature. Get well soon dear mama.

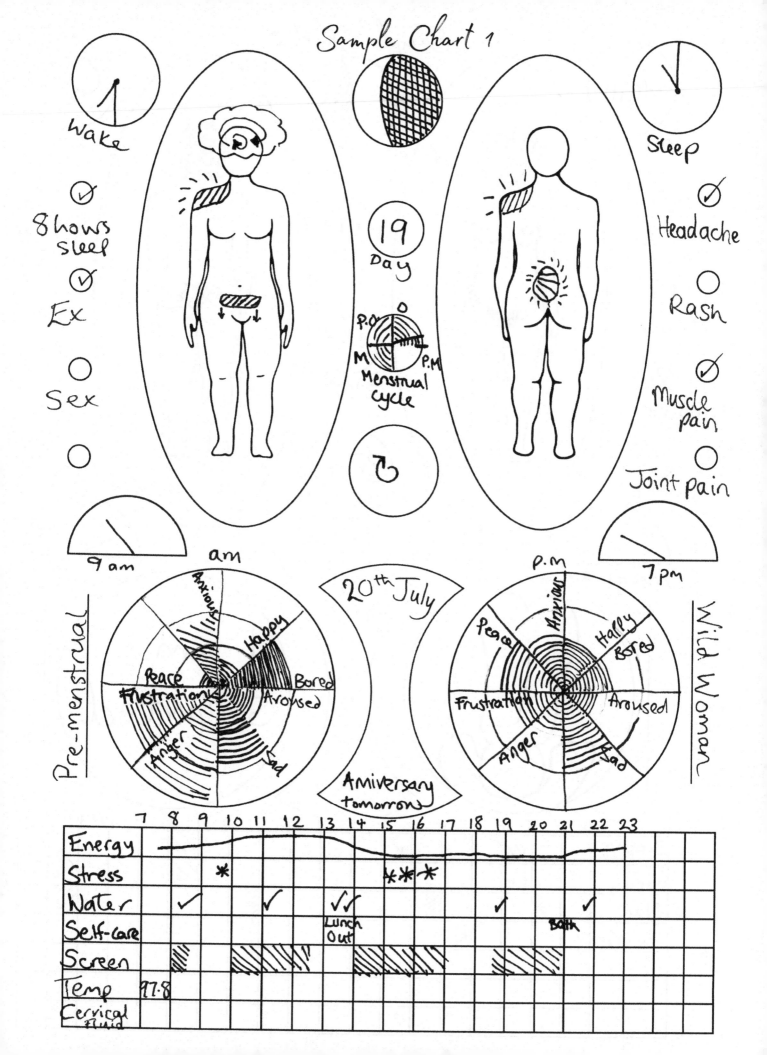

Sample Chart 2

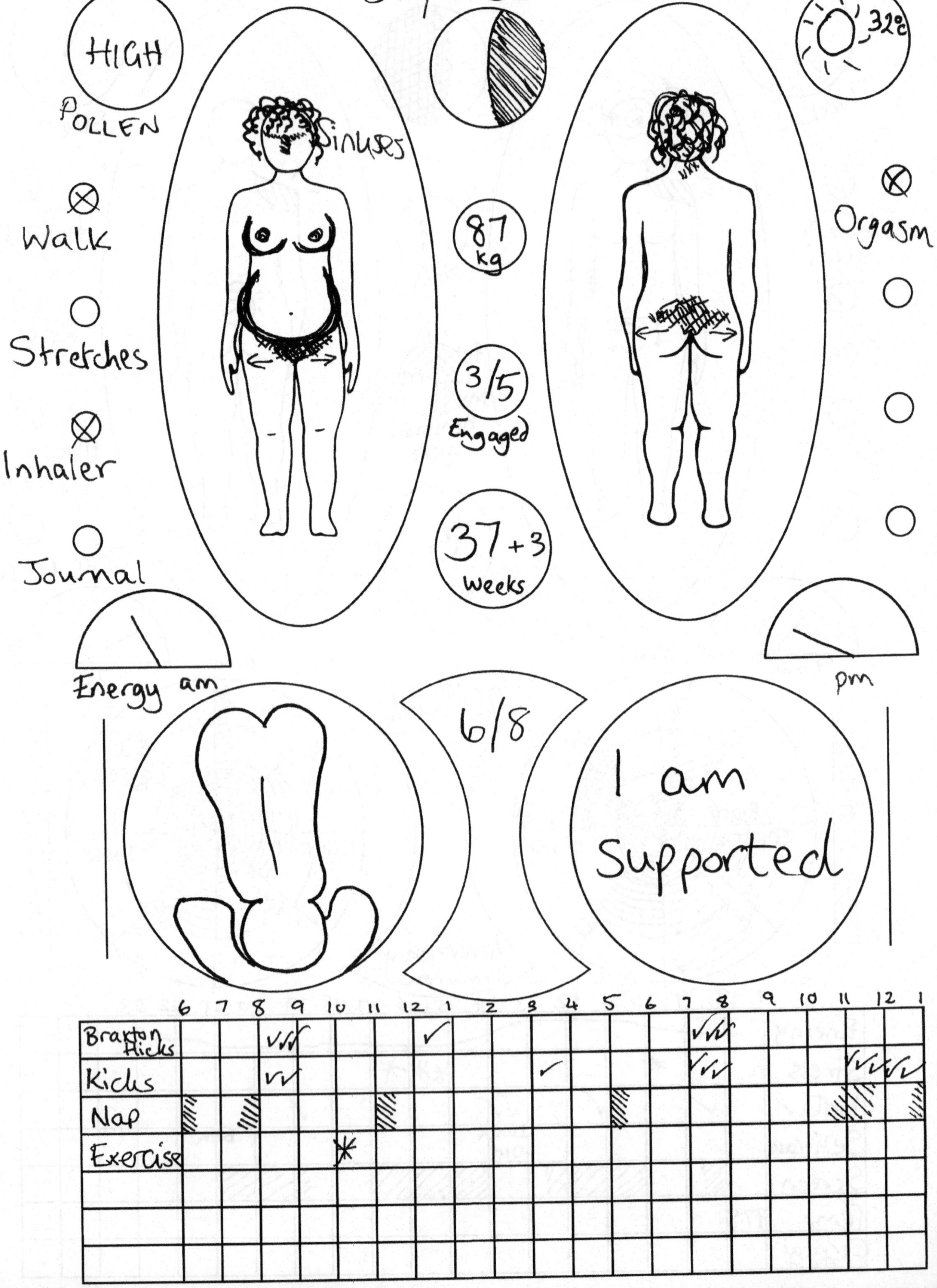

HIGH

POLLEN

⊗ Walk

○ Stretches

⊗ Inhaler

○ Journal

Energy am

87 kg

3/5 Engaged

37+3 weeks

SINUSES

32°C

⊗ Orgasm

○

○

○

pm

6/8

I am supported

	6	7	8	9	10	11	12	1	2	3	4	5	6	7	8	9	10	11	12	1
Braxton Hicks			✓✓✓				✓							✓✓✓						
Kicks			✓✓							✓				✓✓✓				✓✓✓✓		
Nap	▨		▨			▨						▨						▨	▨	
Exercise					✳															

Sample Chart 3

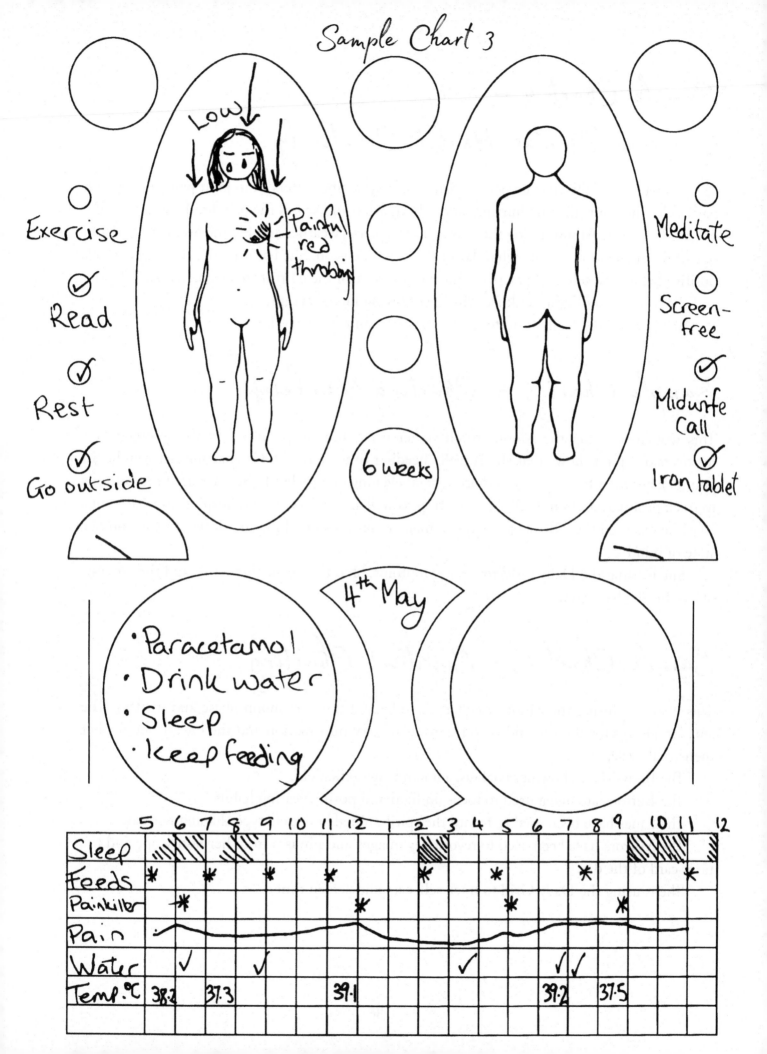

Low

Painful red throbbing

Exercise

☑ Read

☑ Rest

☑ Go outside

6 weeks

Meditate

Screen-free

☑ Midwife Call

☑ Iron tablet

4th May

- Paracetamol
- Drink water
- Sleep
- Keep feeding

	5	6	7	8	9	10	11	12	1	2	3	4	5	6	7	8	9	10	11	12
Sleep		▨	▨	▨						▨								▨	▨	
Feeds	*		*		*		*			*		*			*				*	
Painkiller		*						*				*			*					
Pain																				
Water		✓		✓						✓			✓	✓						
Temp.℃	38.2		37.3				39.1							39.2		37.5				

Sample Chart 4 – Charting Mental Health Creatively

This woman has really enjoyed personalising her pages. She suffers from joint pain and so each day circles the joints that are hurting on the Body Map and scores the pain level out of ten. She has used the large Moons to log the season, moon phase, weather and her introversion level and one of the smaller ones to log what day of her cycle she is on. She has used the Buttons to track positive habits and self-care practices. She has used one of the Mirrors to create her daily doodle and the other to spotlight her knee which is showing lots of symptoms.

She is using the Daily Grid to track symptoms and stress levels.

Sample Chart 5 – Charting Diabetes

This woman is using the Moons to chart her wake and sleep times and the weather. Her introversion spiral shows that she is really needing time alone. She is charting her weight (in pounds), her menstrual cycle and morning and evening energy levels. She has used the Buttons to track positive habits and self-care practices as well as medication and hospital appointments.

She has used the Mirrors as places to make notes on something to ask the doctor, and her state of mind.

She is using the Daily Grid to track symptoms, blood sugar, energy levels and the amount of insulin she has taken.

Sample Chart 6 – Spiritual Charting

This woman is using the Moons to chart the wheel of the year, moon phase and weather. The smaller Moons for the sun and moon signs, planetary information and the lowest one for her menstrual cycle.

The Body Maps show her chakras, aura and energetic field.

The Buttons are being used to focus on food and positive eating habits.

The Lines have been used to record the spirit animal and archetype shaping her day.

The Mirrors have been used to record key images and phrases from her horoscope and the tarot card of the day.

She is using the Daily Grid to track self-care and screen time.

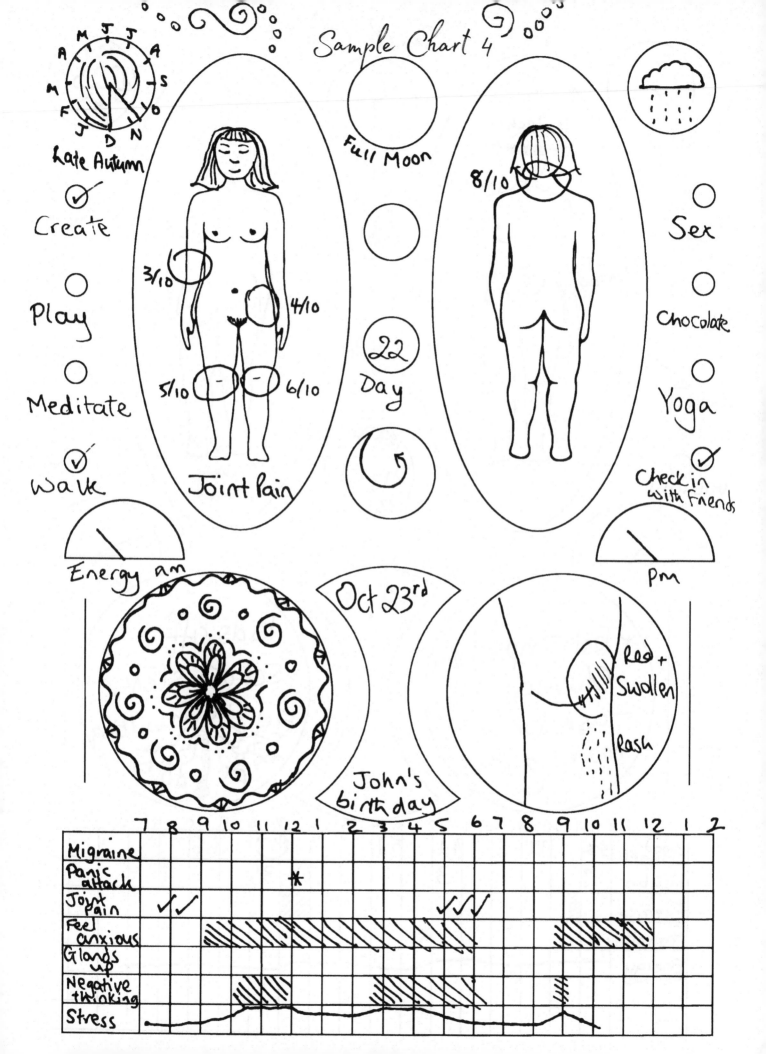

Sample Chart 5

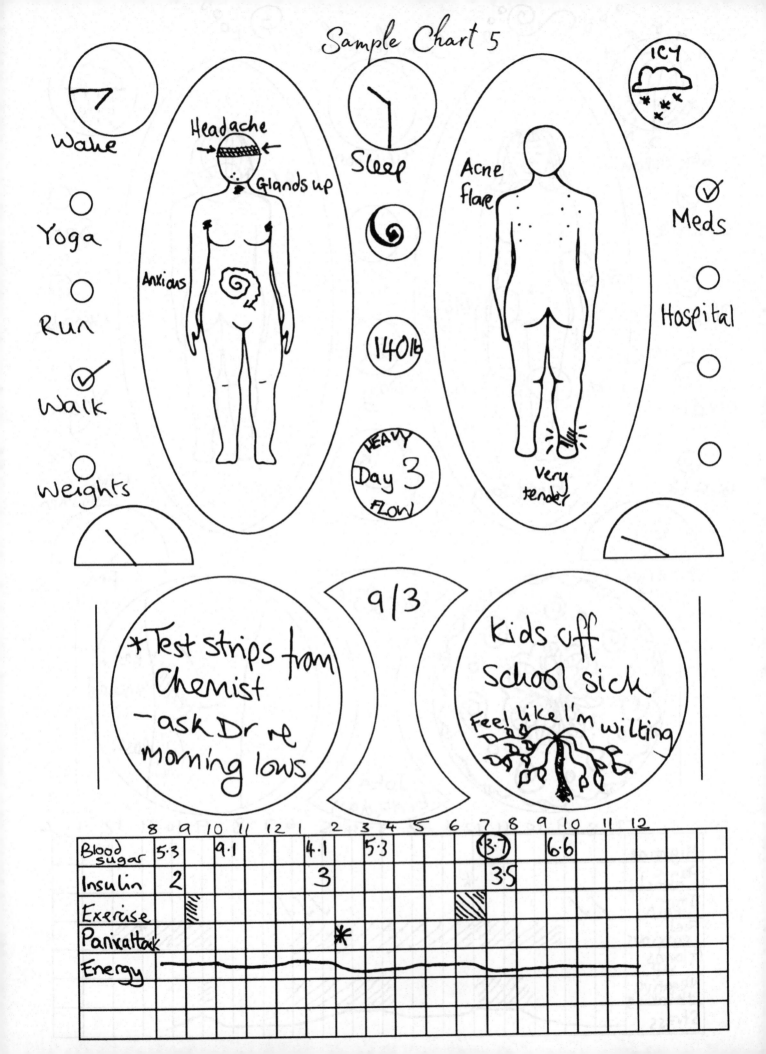

Wake · Yoga · Run · Walk ✓ · Weights

Headache · Glands up · Anxious

Sleep · 140 lb · HEAVY Day 3 FLOW

ICY · ✓ Meds · Hospital

Acne flare · very tender

9/3

* Test strips from Chemist — ask Dr re morning lows

Kids off school sick · Feel like I'm wilting

	8	9	10	11	12	1	2	3	4	5	6	7	8	9	10	11	12
Blood sugar	5.3		9.1			4.1		5.3				(3.7)		6.6			
Insulin	2					3							3.5				
Exercise		▨									▨						
Panic attack							*										
Energy	～～～～～～～～～～～～～～～～																

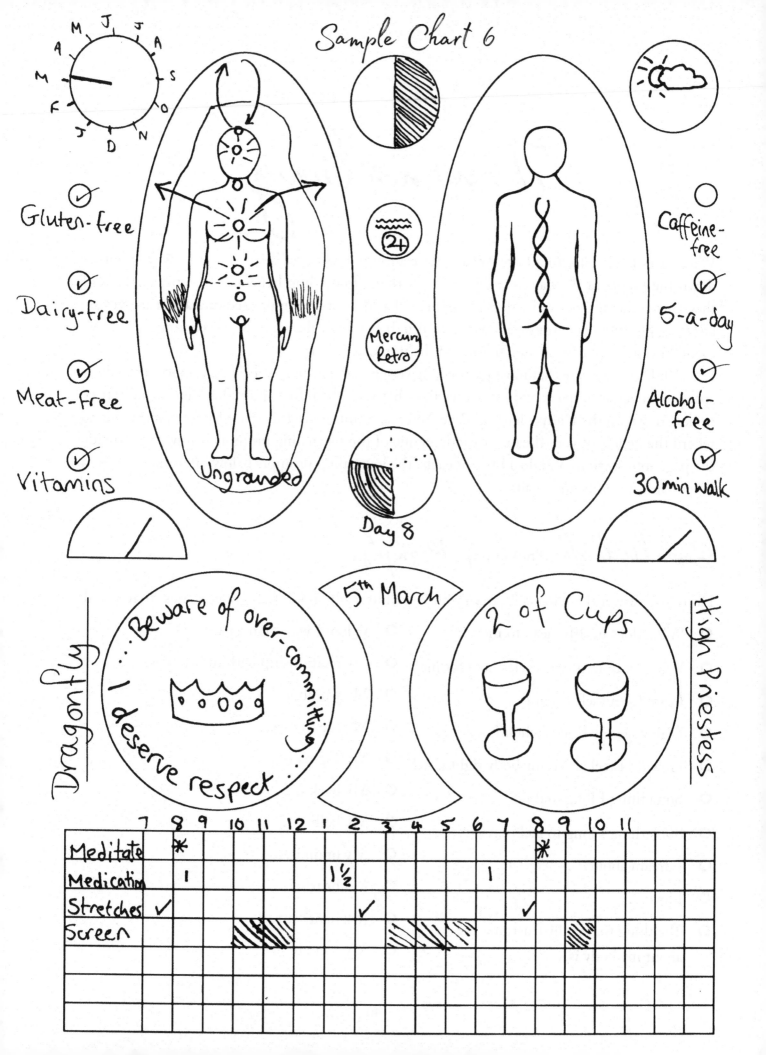

Sample Chart 6

Gluten-free ✓

Dairy-free ✓

Meat-free ✓

Vitamins ✓

Ungrounded

Day 8

Mercury Retro

Caffeine-free ○

5-a-day ✓

Alcohol-free ✓

30 min walk ✓

Dragonfly

Beware of over-committing...
I deserve respect...

5th March

2 of Cups

High Priestess

	7	8	9	10	11	12	1	2	3	4	5	6	7	8	9	10	11
Meditate		✳												✳			
Medication		1					1½						1				
Stretches	✓							✓						✓			
Screen				▨	▨				▨	▨					▨		

Journaling

With every Daily Charting Page you also have a Journaling page. This is not just a way of noting down the events of the day so we don't forget them. Journaling helps us to 'empty our cup' of thoughts and emotions and reflect on them so that they are not repressed or stagnating within, affecting our mood, energy and physical health. It has been shown to positively impact not just mental health, but also the functioning of the immune system.

Whilst I am aware that most of us will have separate journals, I feel it is important to allow space to reflect on, unpack or draw connections between the information that there is only space to note down on the Daily Charting Page. You may want to use this space for free journaling, to record the details of your dreams, to address one of the journaling prompts below, or subdivide the page into sections and do a little of each. The journaling prompts below offer many ways to reflect on your body and health.

Embodied Journaling Prompts

Don't just answer these logically, from your head, but really sink into body awareness to respond.

- What does health mean to me?
- What wisdom do my cycles hold for me?
- I care for myself when I...
- I sabotage my health when I...
- How do I feel about my body right now?
- Something I long to do is...
- Something I long to feel is...
- I dream about...
- I love...
- The thing that really frustrates me about my body is...
- When I was younger I...
- My relationship with my body is...
- My womb is...
- My breasts are...
- My vagina is...
- My back is...
- My belly is...
- My brain is...
- My heart is...
- My hands are...
- My feet are...

- My face is...
- My skin is...
- My hair is...
- My shoulders are...
- My mood is...
- My energy is...
- My breathing is...
- My life is...
- Happiness is...
- I feel...
- When I feel...................
  I...
- If I had a magic wand I would...
- My body is trying to tell me that...
- I am ignoring..............
  because...
- As I get older I am afraid that...
- My heritage means that...
- Something that many in my family
  have struggled with is...
- Being a woman means that...
- I am angry about...
- .... makes me want to cry
  because...
- I am frustrated with...
- I am uncomfortable with...
- When I am angry I...
- I don't want to think about...
- I can't talk about...

- I resent my...
- I am worried about...
- .... does not define me
- I am proud of...
- If I were being honest I would...
- The thing that scares me most is...
- If I were to see my illness as a
  teacher its lesson would be...
- When I am ill I...
- If my body were a place it would be...
- If I were an animal I would be a...
- What best supports my health is...
- My energy is fullest when...
- The thing that scares me most is...
- If my health were more stable I would...
- When I feel calm I...
- What I wish I had known about.......
  was...
- When I am well I...
- I value my...
- Inside I...
- When I am stuck I...
- My mother said...
- I am grateful for my...
- If I imagine my illness as a gift, it
  is giving me...

Monthly Review

The final section of *Full Circle Health* provides a set of tools and exercises to pull together all the precious information you have gathered on a daily basis over the previous month. Use these pages to record and reflect on key goals, achievements, challenges, illnesses and patterns of the month just passed, allowing these insights to inform the coming month ahead.

Monthly Tracker

Use the Monthly Tracker to give you a simple and concise 'at a glance' overview of all your month's information. You can fill it out at the end of the month as a review exercise, or transfer the information from your Daily Charting Pages each day.

- Add the dates (and your cycle days, if using) down the first two columns.

- Then fill in the top boxes with each of the categories you want to track.

- The longer box on the right is for the day's main themes, dreams, archetypes or other notes.

You can easily transfer any of the Button information direct onto the Monthly Tracker. For information that you are taking off the Daily Grid, you will need to find a way of totalling it.

- For example, if you are noting down your water intake, you may choose to total the number of drinks you had in one day – 6 – or the number of millilitres, so 2500ml, if this is important to you.

- Likewise with exercise, you might just want to tick that you exercised that day. Or you may want to fill in the amount of calories burned/steps taken/miles run over the course of the day.

- For sleep you might log the full number of hours slept, how many wakings, quality of sleep rated using a five star system or wake and sleep times.

MONTH: May

Date	Cycle	Wake	Sleep	Stress	Dream Theme
5	1	7.30	(11.30)	*	Loss/change
6	2	(6.00)	(11.45)	(***)	Racing/stress
7	3	8.20	9.40	**	
8	4	9.20	10.30		
9	5	8.45	10.30		
10	6	7.30	9.45	*	
11	7	7.20	10.00		
12	8	(5.00)	9.20	*	High libido
13	9	(6.15)	(12.00)		
14	10	7.00	(1.00)		
15	11	7.20	(11.00)	**	
16	12	(5.20)	(11.15)	(***)	Panic
17	13	6.30	10.30		
18	14	7.10	10.15	*	
19	15	7.00	(11.15)		
20	16	8.20	10.15		
21	17	7.10	10.30	**	Transition-change
22	18	7.20	10.40		
23	19	7.30	(12.00)	*	
24	20	8.25	9.00	(***)	
25	21	7.15	10.30	*	
26	22	(6.00)	10.15		
27	23	8.00	(11.15)	**	Losing things
28	24	8.10	10.00		
29	25	7.50	9.30		End of the world
30	26	8.15	8.45	*	Blood

Habit Tracking

Some habits you may want to track or build include:

- Drinking more water.

- Exercise – for fitness or rehabilitation.

- Meditation/mindfulness/prayer or other spiritual practice.

- Taking medication.

- Coming off medication.

- Food habits like reducing sugar or high cholesterol foods.

- Addictions – noting down when cravings hit, or when you reward yourself – noting down a day without.

- Screen time.

- Early to bed.

- Attending appointments.

You can build in a reward system if you want to and it helps keep you accountable.

Monthly Review

I recommend taking an hour or two at the end of each cycle/month to fill in the Monthly Grid, do a Monthly Review and set goals for the month ahead.

Once you have transferred all the information from your Daily Charting Pages into your Monthly Grid, take some time to look over it. Highlight or circle significant data: any extremes – highs or lows, recurring symptoms or triggers. Reflect on and record the patterns that emerge from this data:

- Can you see any cause/effect relationships? Which events/symptoms cluster? And which show no relationship?

- Which combinations signal health/illness?

- How do cycle days correlate with your health, libido, moods, exercise and creativity?

- What impact do your wake/sleep times have on your energy levels, mood and health?

There are pages to log details of the illnesses you have experienced over the past month, to help you to reflect on and review your health, and others for you to record your achievements. Use the Cycle Circles to log the various cycles that you have been living through over the month and where in each cycle you are now to see if there are any patterns between them.

You can also fill in the second column of your previous Monthly Goals chart.

Monthly Check In

As part of your Monthly Review of data, make time to do your own personal well woman check up. Take a few minutes to look at yourself lovingly in the mirror seeing how your body looks and feels. If you have any injuries or infections, check them. Then take a few moments to:

- Check your physical health such as weight, teeth, breast health...

- Reflect on your predominant mood and energy levels over the course of the last month.

- Focus on the health concerns you have had this month and how you plan to address them in the coming month.

- Note down appointments you need to make for the month ahead.

Goal Setting

As well as tracking and witnessing how your month has gone, it is a great idea to set goals for yourself for the month ahead.

These might include:

- A weekly/daily challenge.

- The amount/type of exercise you intend to do.

- Bedtime or hours sleep you aim at having each night.

- The number of steps you want to walk each day.

- Your calorie intake.

- Vitamins or supplements you intend to take.

- Your goal weight.

- Blood sugar or cholesterol levels.

Diving Deeper

As with all my books, *Full Circle Health* has the potential to be worked on many levels – physical, emotional, spiritual and energetic. You can use this book to simply track your physical and mental health and it will most certainly help you if you want to leave it at this level. If you do, go get started on your charting pages!

This next section is for those who would like to dive deeper into the spiritual and energetic understandings afforded by this system of charting: the metaphysical level. This is how I have used *Full Circle Health* personally, and was my intention behind it.

If I suggest something that does not resonate with you, ask yourself: what about it feels wrong for me? What would be a more acceptable, exciting alternative for me? And then go make it happen. Likewise, if I mention something in passing that intrigues you, explore these 'seed' ideas further – Google them, ask friends and practitioners, question them, find books in the Resources section at the back – try them out in your own life... See if the ideas and activities 'grow corn' for you. Do they work? Do they heal you? Do they help you feel more connected to yourself, and to the people in your life?

Beyond the Physical Body

My understanding of ourselves is as far more than just flesh and bones. Our consciousness, spirit and soul are integral parts of us.

We are complex interconnected systems, embedded within myriad other complex interconnected systems in ways we understand, and many that we still don't. Most of us are only just waking up to this fact, after having been schooled in a mechanical, individualist understanding of nature and our bodies.

Our bodies are always communicating, picking up and processing information on levels other than that which our conscious minds are aware of. Science shows that we communicate not only through speech, but also chemically and energetically. Adrenalin (the stress hormone) and oxytocin (the love hormone) are both 'infectious' – we can pick them up from, and pass them on to others. Our menstrual cycles synchronise hormonally with those of other women when we live in close proximity, as well as with the cycles of the moon. Ideas and feelings, the fruits of consciousness, are contagious. We pass them around via speech, the written word, art, social media and body language. Our dreams and intuition often connect us on a non-material plane with friends, family and teachers. Our bodies and souls have deeper levels of knowing than science currently allows for, with knowledge and memories of things we have not witnessed in person or could not know with our logical minds.

This book cannot possibly track all of the information you receive and the cycles which affect you: you would have no time or brain space left for living if you did! But if you wish, it will help you to become more aware of the interconnections between many of the cycles you experience and increase your ways of knowing, helping you to gain a deeper understanding of your female body and consciousness.

Energy Mapping

Energy is a precursor to thought, feeling and action. It provides the building blocks of the physical, material world.

But most of us were taught little if anything about the energy in our bodies and how it shifts. Western science tends to dismiss that which it cannot currently measure. Our energy is one of those things. We can only define it with words – *I'm feeling wobbly, I'm feeling blocked, I'm feeling flat, I'm scared to death, I'm exhilarated*. We can measure a person's heart rate, temperature, levels of brain activity, we can observe behaviour and whether they are flushed or pale, but not their energy field, not what is going on under the surface, on the next level down.

Our culture tends to teach us to ignore – or be scared of – anything that cannot be seen or defined physically. This is certainly true when it comes to energy.

But many other cultures have a well-established and clearly mapped understanding of energy in the body, as firmly believed in as the blood or reproductive systems. These include *chi* from ancient Chinese medicine, *prana*, *kundalini* and the chakra system from yogic thought, energy defences and auras in New Age healing as well as other systems of thought from native cultures around the world used by shamans, wise women and traditional healers.

Energy is understood in these traditions as underlying all aspects of our physical and mental health, our creativity, libido, fertility… When our energy is low, stagnated or blocked we experience certain symptoms or diseases depending on where in the body is blocked and the severity. Over-active energy can also cause ill health, and so the approach is to harmonise or balance the individual's internal energy system and external energy field. The individual energy system is also seen as being deeply integrated with the energy systems of the Earth, other species, the planets and stars, and it is understood that shifts in any of these affect each of us.

If these approaches resonate with you, then please know that this book has been designed to support your growing awareness, to enable you to integrate it into your understanding of your own health. I need to stress that I am not a trained energy worker in any discipline but have a life-long interest in it, from my own healing journey, my work and research to do with it. If you are wanting to build your understanding of this topic, I have included several very useful books in the Resources section.

As women we have particularly dynamic bodies and energy which shifts powerfully during our menstrual cycles, sexual arousal, if we are pregnant, post-partum or breastfeeding or going through menopause. This is on top of the mental health and energetic and health shifts that all humans experience. We are dynamic, and we are supposed to be. This is healthy. But as women we are taught little about the cycles of our shifting energy.

Energy, whilst invisible to most of us, has certain qualities that can be perceived using the other ways of knowing that I discussed earlier. It has an intensity or frequency, and usually a direction and quality. Energy tends towards flow and stagnates when blocked. If you get into the habit of being aware of your life-force energy: its source, intensity and direction, this helps hugely in enabling you to keep it flowing through you (and you through it), and to address blockages, stagnation, and excess energy.

How do you know what your energy is doing? You use your inner senses – your intuition, inner eye, as well as body feeling. It takes practice. But is an important skill to have. Because once you are aware of the energy then you can learn to express it healthily. You are aware of the feeling of a downward spiral, or an upward one. You are aware if it is fast or slow in its onset.

When starting out understanding your energy, focus on these questions:

- O Where do I feel it in my body?

- O What quality does it have?

- O How intense is it? Is it increasing or decreasing in intensity?

- O How do I respond? What does it make me do/want to do?

- O What does it remind me of that I have experienced before?

- O What metaphors describe it best? What colour/image/words come with it?

- O How long does it last?

- O Is it coming from the inside… or the outside?

- O What happens if I ignore it? What happens if I respond to it?

- O What might it be trying to tell me?

- O How can I express it best?

- O Does it make me feel uncomfortable? Why might this be?

- O Who in my life can help support me with this if it feels too big to manage alone?

- O What has sparked it? When did it start?

Get into the habit of knowing where your energy is 'at' and where your mental attention is too. Often our mental energy is in our head, or drifting off outside of us, meanwhile our physical energy is absorbed elsewhere in our bodies. What we are trying to do is to bring our awareness out of our heads and into our bodies and connect it with our physical energy. The first thing you will be doing when you chart is to observe what is happening with your energy. Blocked energy may manifest as: feelings of lethargy, constant anger, low mood or depression, thoughts racing round in circles becoming fixations and paranoia, feeling creatively or spiritually stuck or blocked, having no libido. All of these are perfectly normal parts of our life experiences, however we usually feel them deeply and then move through them. When we struggle to move on and become stuck in them, when they come to dominate our lives and health then they become problematic. This is where the next step comes in: learning to shift blockages within your energetic system and maintain and support the dynamic flow of energy. You can do this by using the Buttons to set goals or daily reminders for yourself.

Take a moment to reflect: what do you do to unblock your energy? Possibilities include:

O	Talk with someone	O	Meditation or mindfulness
O	Scream into a pillow	O	Laugh
O	Dance	O	Aromatherapy
O	A brisk walk or run	O	Read
O	A bath or shower	O	Get out in nature
O	Sex or masturbation	O	See a therapist or counsellor
O	Sing	O	....
O	Create something	O	....
O	Journal	O	....
O	Massage or bodywork	O	....
O	Energy work, such as reiki	O	....
O	Prayer	O	....

Tick off those that help you, and add more. Pick your top six, and allocate them daily Buttons. If you are someone who tends to get energetically stuck, these daily reminders can be a real help.

Your Energetic Field

You will notice that the Body Map is contained within an oval. This shape is meant to be both a reminder of our energy or aura, but also of our energetic boundaries, a visual reminder of what lies within your sphere of influence, your physical and energetic world... and what is outside. Now, of course, these are blurred in many ways, but for those of us who are empathic or highly sensitive, or who struggle with boundary issues, this visual reminder to differentiate between the inner and outer world, and our ability to strengthen our boundaries in order to contain our own energy to keep ourselves physically and emotionally safe, is an important one.

You might choose to colour the space between the body and the oval to reflect the colours in your aura, or to reflect what your energy field contains. Then you can write around the outside of the oval people and events that are significantly affecting your health and energy. You might use arrows or lines to represent energy cords that are intruding through your energy boundaries, and where they are affecting your body. For example are they 'taking up your headspace', 'pulling on your heartstrings' or do you feel you have just been 'punched in the guts'? What do these metaphors look and feel like in your body? And how might this insight help you heal their impact?

You may choose to include your seven chakras on the figure, if this is something that you work with. Perhaps tune into each of these and colour them large or small depending on how the energy is flowing through them, how connected they feel, whether some feel blocked or shut down.

If chakras are new to you, a simple way to describe them is being like wheels or gates that our energy runs through. Each chakra is represented by a colour. These are analogous to the colours of the rainbow, and start at the base or root chakra, with red, going through the colours of the rainbow, orange in the womb area, yellow at the solar plexus, green in the heart, blue in the throat, indigo at the third eye and violet at the crown.

What is important to remember is that filling in this diagram is like taking an energetic snapshot of your body and noting all the things that you cannot see – physical and energetic – at one point in your day. But your energy is dynamic and ever-changing. If you want a more continuous way of tracking your energy, you may choose to use one line of the Daily Grid to create a rough line graph of your energy levels throughout the day.

Menstrual Charting

If you have never charted your menstrual cycle before you may be wondering why you should! Short of knowing when to have sanitary protection ready, many women live pretty much oblivious to where in their cycle they are.

For about four decades, unless you are pregnant, breastfeeding, using hormonal birth control or without a womb or cycles, every single day of most women's lives is situated somewhere on the menstrual cycle. Whether ovulating or bleeding, struggling with PMS or conception, our bodies, our energy levels, our sense of self, even our abilities are constantly changing each and every day. Our cycles impact our mental health, our pain thresholds, even our susceptibility to infection.

And yet we rarely talk about it.

Women are expected to be the same, day in, day out. Despite the fact that our bodies are changing hormonally from one day to the next. Charting helps to keep track of where you are in your cycle and gives a frame of reference for symptoms you may be experiencing.

Most of us were not taught about the experiential aspects of our cycles, let alone the spiritual and intuitive gifts of menstruation, or the way that menstruation impacts our dreams. I am sharing the integrated menstrual chart I created for my book *Moon Time: harness the ever-changing energy of your menstrual cycle,* to give you a basic overview of the effects of the cycle on your mood, energy and physical health.

If you are doing any form of fertility charting such as the Billings or Sympto-Thermal Method of Natural Family Planning you may choose to dedicate some of your Daily Grid or Moon spaces to logging your cervical fluid, cervical position and morning temperature alongside your basic cycle-tracking information and unprotected male-female sexual intercourse, so that you have all of your information in one place.

When logging your cycle you can create a Cycle Circle by subdividing one of the larger Moons into rough quadrants corresponding to the four major phases – menstrual, pre-ovulatory, ovulatory and pre-menstrual. Or you can, if you have a regular cycle and know exactly how many days you are, note down the right amount of days on the circle – like minutes on a clock – and point the clock hand at the correct day. You may also just choose to write the day of your cycle down in a smaller Moon, where Day 1 corresponds to the first day of your bleeding, and then each day after is counted until the first day of your next period, which is Day 1 of a new cycle.

	PRE-OVULATORY	OVULATORY
MOON PHASE	Waxing	Full
ARCHETYPE	Virgin/Maiden	Mother
SEASON	Spring	Summer
ELEMENT	Air	Earth
LIGHT	Lightening	Full bright light
LENGTH	9 days	5 days
HORMONE	Oestrogen	Rising oestrogen and progesterone.
PHYSICAL	Egg follicle ripening – stimulating breast and womb.	Egg released from ovary into fallopian tube, becomes *corpus luteum*. Uterine wall built up in preparation for fertilisation.
VAGINAL DISCHARGE	Sticky/none	Clear and stretchy, like egg white. Very wet feeling.
EMOTION	Calm, open, dynamic, clear, energetic, enthusiastic, able to cope with irritations.	Loving, nurturing, nourishing, sustaining, energised, connected.
ENERGY	Rising dynamic – growing outward.	Full, sustaining – losing sense of self in work or mothering.
LIBIDO	Rising, carefree.	Full, horny, height of libidinous desire around full moon/ovulation.
PHYSICAL FEELING	Energetic	Perhaps ovulatory pain/cramping, sometimes mid-cycle spotting, food cravings, horny, sensitive breasts.
OUTWARD ACTION	Start projects – clear visioning and energy raising. Fresh start. Organise and prioritise. Clear out – spring cleaning. Catch up with things that have slipped during menstruation.	Work hard, love well – birth creative projects, stay up late! Harmony with nature and other mothers. Receptive to others' input.
RELATION-SHIPS	Easy-going, trusting, out-going.	Loving, giving, nurturing. Reach out to friends, children, family and partner.
KEY WORDS	New beginnings, dynamic, exuberance, self-confident.	Fertility, radiating, caring, nurturing, committed.
AFFIRMATION	I step forward in action with a lightness of heart.	I embrace my life with love and generate beauty around me.

PRE-MENSTRUAL	MENSTRUAL
Waning	Dark
Enchantress/Wild Woman	Crone/Wise Woman
Autumn	Winter
Fire	Water
Darkening	Dark
9 days	5 days
Falling oestrogen and progesterone.	Progesterone
Transition time.	Womb lining breaks down and released from uterus.
None/blobby, thick and yellow	Bleeding – starting out bright red, becoming browner towards the end.
Creative, emotional, sensitive, angry.	Introspective, dreamy, sensitive, intuitive, spiritually connected.
Waning dynamic – destructive, descending inward.	Reflective, slow, containing, internalised, spiritual.
Peaks and troughs – can be very intense.	Often a sexual peak just before bleeding occurs, or just after. Little desire during menstruation.
Lowered immune system. Towards the end: cramping, back ache, bloating, tiredness, tender breasts, sugar and carbohydrate cravings, hostility, mood swings.	Greater need for rest and dreaming sleep. Cramping, back ache, migraine, faintness, exhaustion, tearfulness.
Finish up projects. Begin to reflect and assess. Take action dealing with issues and problems. Turn your focus to inner-directed creative projects and listen deeply to your intuition.	Retreat, dream time. Only do what is essential. Do not take on any new projects. Delay important decisions or stressful appointments. Slow down, tune in deeply to your intuition and rest well.
Needs to balance dynamic interactions with others, with focused, energised creative time alone.	Desires to be alone or in quiet communion with other women – does not want to be around men and children!
Magical, witchy, destructive, intuitive.	Darkness, wisdom, gestation, stillness, vision.
I use the sword of my intolerance to cut deep and true. I keep hold of my vision and manifest it.	I sink into my depths and listen to my dreams.

Phases of the Moon

Charting the phases of the moon may also be new to you. Why do we do it?

Myriad cultures around the world have been organised around lunar calendars, but ours is solar. The moon is understood to have a significant impact on many life forms, including humans. Physically it would be strange if it did not affect us, bearing in mind its gravitational pull controls the world's tidal patterns, and our bodies are made up of 70% water. Its changing brightness impacts our internal hormonal balance and wake/sleep cycles and has been observed by many cultures to affect our energy, dreams, healing and intuitive abilities. Many professionals attest to the very real influence of the moon on human behaviour in their work. Teachers will tell you that their students are more unruly and 'wired' at full moon. Casualty admissions often spike. Midwives are aware that the full moon seems to trigger labour in many pregnant women and current research shows an increase in schizophrenic and epileptic episodes at full moon time – behaviour previously referred to as 'lunatic'.

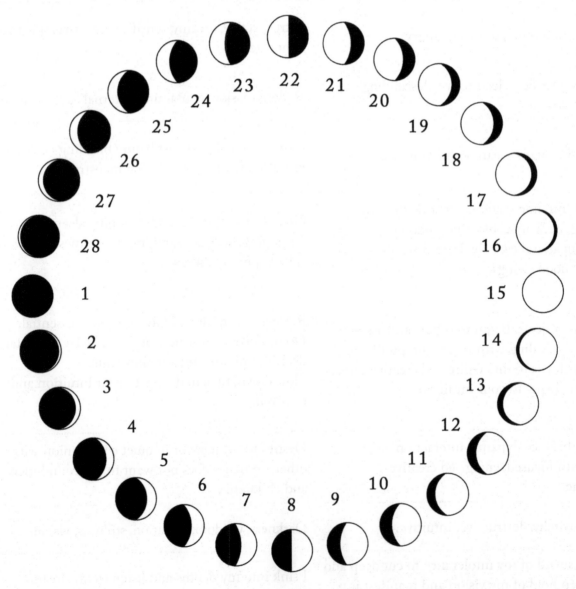

In spiritual terms the moon with its constantly changing face is associated with feminine consciousness, whereas the sun is associated with the masculine. Many women find that learning more about, and integrating the moon's phases into their lives, has a profoundly positive effect in understanding their changing energies, menstrual cycles and moods. The connection between the moon and menstrual cycles has been observed since the dawn of human history. The average 28-day menstrual cycle correlates closely with the moon's cycle, and women's cycles often synchronise not only with each other, but also with the moon. But even if you don't have cycles, the moon impacts your sleep. It has been shown that the full moon has a strong negative impact on the quality of sleep, regardless of whether the moon is visible or not.

If you choose to chart the moon phases, the easiest way is by filling in one of the Moons to correspond to its current phase. To learn more about the moon's phases, make a conscious effort to check the sky every day, check the phases online or on a calendar. The following is a simplified version of the moon's phases and the energetic properties of each.

Full Moon

Full moons rise at sunset and set at dawn. This is the time when the moon's pull is at its strongest, meaning higher tides. Full moons are usually experienced as full of energy – sometimes in a good way, and others creating agitation, making sleep and relaxation hard. Full moons are a time to harvest and sow, a time to entertain and celebrate, to work late and create wholeheartedly. Each full moon has its own special name and characteristics.

Waning Moon

Waning means getting smaller. When the moon reaches its halfway point (the last quarter moon, which rises around midnight) there is a sense of balance, tension or transition. It continues getting smaller each night, until it is completely dark.

The Dark or New Moon

For a couple of days the moon is almost invisible, it is a time of darkness. The moon is in shadow and rises before dawn and sets with the sun. Many traditions use this as a time of inwardness, reflection, visioning and setting intentions for the month ahead. It is a time of new beginnings, a seeming pause in the darkness before its journey back to fullness again. In terms of tides, its effect is equal to that of the full moon.

Waxing Moon

The moon gets a little bigger and brighter each night, moving through the *crescent* moon – the moon of story-books, the small sliver which speaks of hope, new life, magic. When it reaches halfway (the first quarter) again there is a sense of transition or balance.

Thresholds and Transitions

Cycles tend to have power points – places where the energy is higher, where we feel good and powerful. They also have pressure points, times when we are challenged, when we experience internal or external pressure and find ourselves struggling.

It was Penelope Shuttle who first drew my attention to the importance of the threshold times of our menstrual cycles – the crossing points between phases: premenstrual to menstrual and ovulatory to premenstrual being the most obvious. These are places where our bodies are in transition between states of being: our hormones are shifting, and we are emotionally more volatile, energetically more chaotic and physically more vulnerable to infection.

I began to notice that these transition points in my life are where the greatest potential for big change occurs, as if they are power points or physical 'chakras' that we pass through. Often they mark the 'beginning/end' point of a cycle. Each has the potential for positive or negative change and strong emotion. It has the potential to be a 'power' point or a 'pressure' point depending on our health, energy levels and attitude. Thresholds include:

- Birth/death.
- Waking/falling asleep.
- The end of one cycle of time – a day, week, month or year and the beginning of a new one.
- Birthdays and anniversaries.
- Dark/full moon.
- Beginning or end of a diet or exercise regime.
- Beginning or end of medication or therapeutic treatment.
- Beginning or end of a job or relationship.
- Time away from daily routine.

Find time to slow your life down at these points, pay attention and take extra care of yourself. Know that you will be more energetically charged, and perhaps physically and emotionally stressed at these times. But know too that the opportunity for deep transformative experiences also lies within these threshold places. Note down your key power and pressure points:

Power Points   *Pressure Points*

Dissonance and Flow

What you will notice is that these various cycles correlate – the energy of the waxing moon corresponds to spring time, a phase of growth and budding and bloom. It also corresponds to the Maiden archetype representing pre-ovulation in the menstrual cycle. There is a sense of the energy being fresh, young, vibrant and building.

Midsummer corresponds to the full moon, the Mother archetype and ovulation. This is a time of fullness, abundance, high energy and fertility. We find ourselves extroverted, nurturing, creative and fully engaged with the world around us.

Autumn brings with it a turning inwards, the wild winds that shake the trees are represented by tempestuous shifting moods of the pre-menstrual phase, shown in the archetype of the Wild Woman. This is a time of preparing to shed the old, to put harvest to store, and prepare for winter.

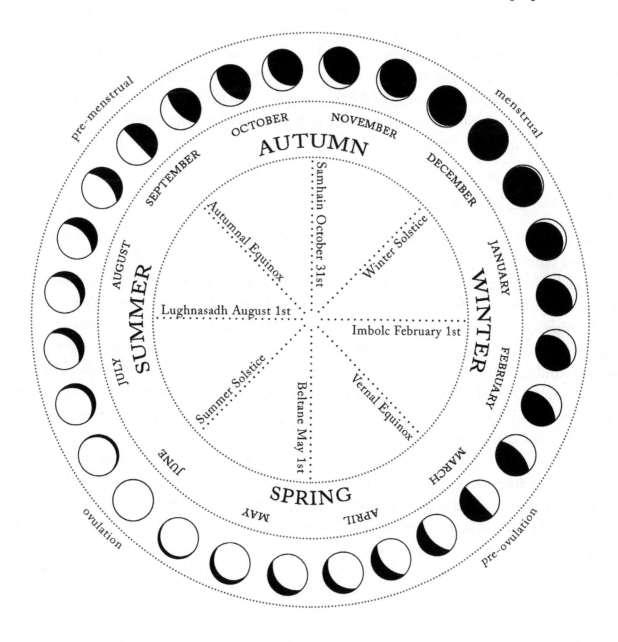

Winter brings hibernation, we rest in our caves away from the world and are at our most fully introverted. This is represented by the Crone, the dark moon. This is a powerful energy, when our wisdom is drawn within ourselves. It is a time of reflection and rest, and the kindling of new potential within the darkness. It marks a time of grief and relief that comes with death and release of the old, and offers the void space of infinite possibility.

When all the cycles align like this, we can feel a deep sense of 'rightness', as our bodies cycles are in harmony with the cycles around us. This is known as 'flow' and represents a state of healthy dynamic balance. Whereas when our bodies and the cycles beyond us are diametrically opposed – for example, being pre-menstrual in the spring, or bleeding on the full moon, or forced to be busy and extroverted during the winter holidays when we are menstruating, we really feel the energetic dissonance, and without conscious awareness of this can be confused as to why we feel so out of sorts.

Often when we feel this way our physical or mental health can go out of balance, mood swings become stronger, and we can try to compensate using familiar crutches: alcohol, carbohydrates, over eating, starving ourselves, medication, or other ways of numbing ourselves physically and emotionally in order to get through the day. When we find ourselves drained because of the dissonance of cycles, we can tend to turn to easy energy boosts: coffee, stimulants, chocolate, sugar to put us 'back on our game'. Whilst these might seem to work in the short term, each can cause dependency, a build up of toxins in our system, and systemic exhaustion as we ignore our bodies' natural signals of tiredness, leading to burn out and more serious ill health.

Dream Charting

Our dreams act as a bridge between our days, between our conscious and unconscious minds, inner and outer worlds, spiritual and material realms. Our emotions, medication, sexuality, the moon and what is going on in the outside world all have a direct impact on our dream lives. Dreams also alter according to our menstrual cycles – certain images and archetypes emerge at specific times in our cycle, and ovulation often leads to erotic dreams. Our dreams are affected hugely by our waking mental states – when we are anxious we can often spend nights running for buses and trains, or losing our children. When trauma is activated in our bodies nightmares tend to haunt our nights. When we are pregnant we may dream of birthing or conversing with our unborn child. Dreams can be pre-cognitive, prophetic, bring us omens, warnings, teachings or insight into big life transitions.

In many native cultures women are known as the dreamers for their tribes and their ability to connect to the ancestors and Dream World are considered powerful important gifts. Ceremonies and dream lodges are held at new moons and during menstruation where their dreams are shared in circle and their wisdom gathered to assist the community.

Charting our dreams – writing down what we remember of them as soon as we awaken and working with dream images – can give profound insight into the crossovers between our bodies, conscious minds and our subconscious world. Often when reflecting on these dreams we can find wisdom for our waking lives.

The more we get into the habit of charting our dreams, the easier they become to recall. You may want to record the following:

- Key dream images – places, characters, themes that recur, develop or progress over the course of the month. Be sure to record the dream verbatim before recording your analysis or interpretation.

- Themes that recur on a monthly basis in the same lunar, menstrual or astrological phase.

- How your dreams reflect your inner and outer life.

- How your dreams impact your waking mood.

- Interactions between your libido, creativity, spiritual life, dream life and physical or mental health.

Charting the Spirit

Astrology has been used by cultures around the world to gain insight into current and future events. Whether your understanding of astrology is as rudimentary as checking your horoscope occasionally, or you are learned in the transits of the planets, and fluent in your north node lunar sign you can use the charting pages to log these insights too.

Archetypes are another way of gaining insight into our consciousness, health and growth. You may choose to note the menstrual archetype that is dominant each day – Maiden when you are pre-ovulatory, Mother during ovulation, Wild Woman during the premenstrual phase and Crone during menstruation. You may also have a felt sense of the archetype dominating your life at present – the Wise Woman, Teacher, Student, Fool… You can do this intuitively or pull an archetype or tarot card.

The sky is the limit in charting the influences of key aspects of your belief system: festivals, holy days, feast days; the rune or ogham for the day; spirit guides, saints, goddesses or angels which you are invoking that day; the predominant element or position on the medicine wheel.

Circle Charting

Circle charting is a common tool amongst wise women. It can be used to chart the menstrual cycle and/or dreams along with lunar and astrological information. Penelope Shuttle in *Alchemy for Women*, Connie Cockrell Kaplan in *The Woman's Book of Dreams: dreaming as a spiritual practice*, Patrícia Lemos and Ana Afonso in *The Goddess in You* and Zoe Shekinah's moon dial mandala all use circle charting technology. I love the aesthetics and symbolism, not to mention the simple elegance of having all the information on one circle, however, personally I find the format quite crowded to use. But this book is called *Full Circle Health*, so it would be remiss to leave it out.

At the end of your Monthly Review Pages you will find two Full Circle Charts - one subdivided into 30 like the one below, and one blank for you to use for months or cycles longer than 30 days. Around the outer rim fill in the date and your cycle day. You can also fill in the sign which the moon is in. For each day fill in either the menstrual symptoms you are tracking, or the main images or themes from your dream.

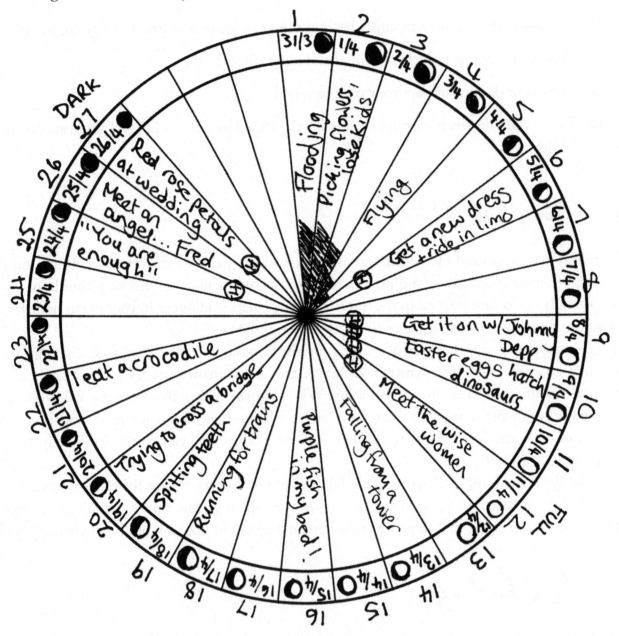

In this example, the days of the menstrual cycle have been noted around the outside of the circle, and in the inner rim are the day's date and moon phases. The wedges are used to record key images and themes from dreams and the inside of the circle logs the heaviness of bleeding (shading on days 1-5) and an H in a circle denotes days of high libido.

Coming Full Circle

As we begin to consciously experience all the cycles that our bodies are immersed in, we learn the wisdom of the circle in an embodied manner. We understand that the end of one cycle is always the beginning of another. Cycles remind us that everything has its time, its own rhythm, and that forcing causes suffering, and rarely makes anything change for the better. The cycle teaches us the wisdom of the body – that rhythm is health.

Each cycle we have the opportunity to learn a little more, or a little more deeply...
Each cycle we are asked:

- To move more deeply into both the known and the unknown.
- To let go of the old.
- To walk into the void with courage.
- To deal with repetition with curiosity, gratitude and patience.
- To reflect on what we have learned during the last cycle, and apply that wisdom to the new cycle... leaving space for our not knowing, for the newness as it emerges.

As you become more aware of the various cycles you are engaged in, you may want to reflect in the journaling pages:

- What cycles seem to be repeating?
- What cycles are you immersed in?
- Where in each cycle are you?
- What does it mean to come full circle?
- How might you mark or celebrate this with a ritual or reflection?
- How can you integrate the wisdom you have acquired during the previous cycle?

When I was creating this book I used it to chart my way through a whole menstrual cycle in order to become more consciously aware of the feminine in my physical body, moods, energy levels and consciousness. It was when I got to the end of my menstrual month that the title of the book came to me – *Full Circle Health*. I had experienced viscerally the sense of coming full circle in my own life, in a way that I had not experienced so fully before, despite having charted my cycle for years. I was immersed in my own self. I could see patterns that had previously eluded me. Once I had come full circle, I started all over again, eager to be able to see how one menstrual month compared to the next in terms of my creativity, libido, dreams and energy levels. Finally I had a tool that helped me to really see myself.

My dearest wish is that this will be a powerful tool for you too, helping to initiate you more deeply into the wisdom inherent in your female body and consciousness. I am honoured to play a part in holding space for their powerful emergence and your vibrant health.

Resources

Planners, Diaries and other charting resources

Full Circle Health: 3-month charting journal – Lucy H. Pearce

Full Circle Health printable charting pages – shop.womancraftpublishing.com

Moon Dreams: charting diary – Starr Meneely

The Goddess in You – Patrícia Lemos and Ana Afonso

We'Moon Diary – Mother Tongue Ink

Earth Pathways Diary

My Shining Year – Life Planner – Leonie Dawson

Moon Dial Mandala – shop.womancraftpublishing.com

Women's Health

Moon Time: harness the ever-changing energy of your menstrual cycle – Lucy H. Pearce

Medicine Woman – Lucy H. Pearce

Moods of Motherhood: the inner journey of mothering – Lucy H. Pearce

Women's Bodies, Women's Wisdom – Dr Christiane Northrup

Woman Heal Thyself: an ancient healing system for contemporary women
  – Jeanne Elizabeth Blumm

Our Bodies, Ourselves – Boston Women's Health Cooperative

Taking Charge of your Fertility – Toni Weschler

Alchemy for Women: personal transformation through dreams and the female cycle
  – Penelope Shuttle and Peter Redgrove

Red Moon: understanding and using the creative, sexual and spiritual gifts of the menstrual cycle
  – Miranda Gray

Wild Power: Discover the Magic of Your Menstrual Cycle and Awaken the Feminine Path to Power
  – Sjanie Hugo Wurlitzer and Alexandra Pope

Fully Conscious Woman (YouTube) – Jane Hardwicke Collings

The Hormone Cure: reclaim balance, sleep, sex drive and vitality naturally with the Gottfried protocol
  – Dr Sara Gottfried

Mood Mapping: plot your way to emotional health and happiness – Dr Liz Miller

Shining Academy – Leonie Dawson – Habit Tracker

Thirteen Moons – Rachael Hertogs

Circle Wisdom

Mother Rising: the blessingway journey into motherhood—Cortlund, Lucke & Watelet

Circle of Stones – Judith Duerk

The Circle is Sacred: a medicine book for women – Scout Cloud Lee

Sacred Circles: a guide to creating your own women's spirituality group
  – Robin Cairns and Sally Craig

The Women's Wheel of Life: 13 archetypes of woman at her fullest power – Elizabeth Davis

Birthing Ourselves into Being – Baraka Elihu

Energy and Healing

The Rainbow Way: cultivating creativity in the midst of motherhood – Lucy H. Pearce

Energy Anatomy: the science of personal power, spirituality and health
  – Caroline Myss (audio)

Anatomy of the Spirit: the seven stages of power and healing – Caroline Myss

Hands of Light: a guide to healing through the human energy field – Barbara Ann Brennan

Eastern Body, Western Mind: psychology and the chakra system as a path to the self
  – Anodea Judith

Energy Medicine for Women: aligning your body's energies to boost your health and vitality
  – Donna Eden

The Highly Sensitive Person: how to thrive when the world overwhelms you – Elaine Aron

Dancing the Dream: the seven sacred paths of human transformation – Jamie Sams

Why People Don't Heal (YouTube) – Caroline Myss

Wild Feminine: finding power, spirit and joy in the female body – Tami Lynn Kent

Art is a Way of Knowing – Pat B. Allen

You Can Heal Your Life – Louise. L. Hay

The Woman's Book of Dreams: dreaming as a spiritual practice – Connie Cockrell Kaplan

My Daily Charting Pages

My intentions and goals for this month...

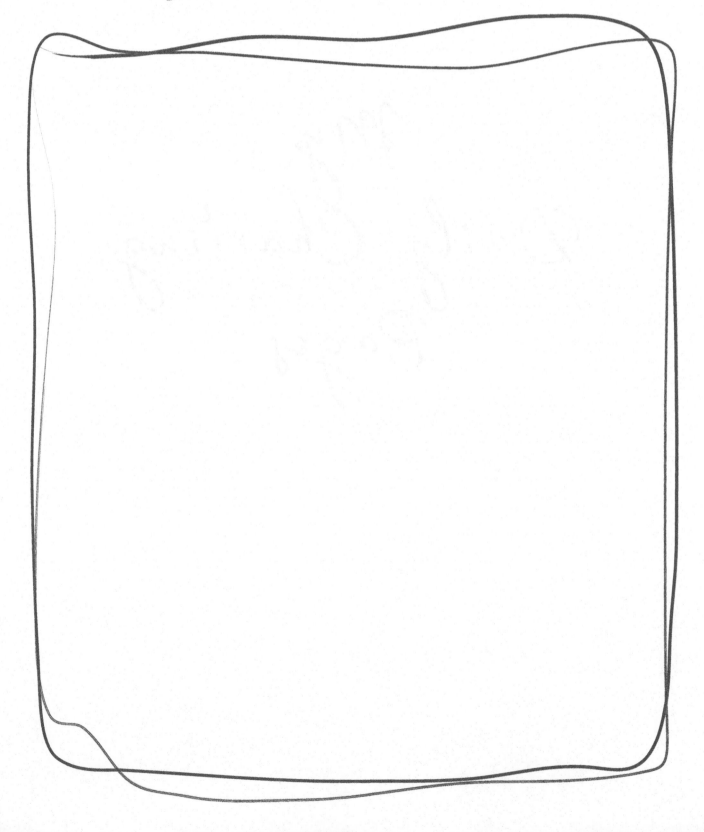

Charting Key

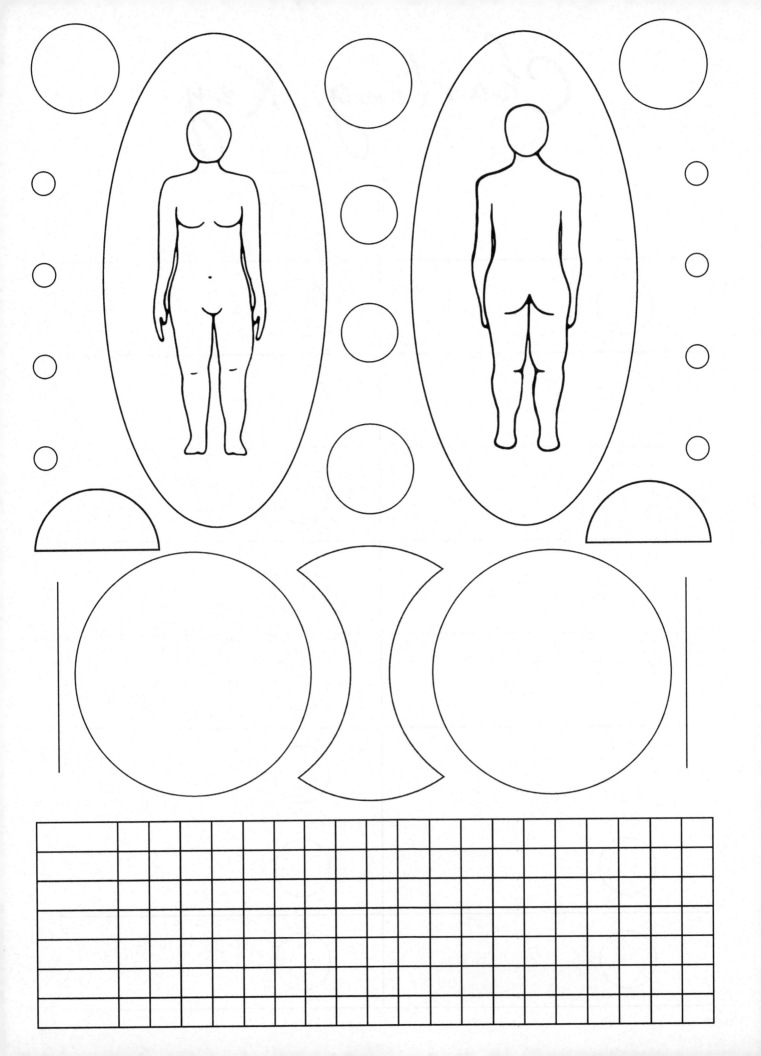

I need... I dreamed... I am... I feel... I hope... I am worried about... I am thankful for...

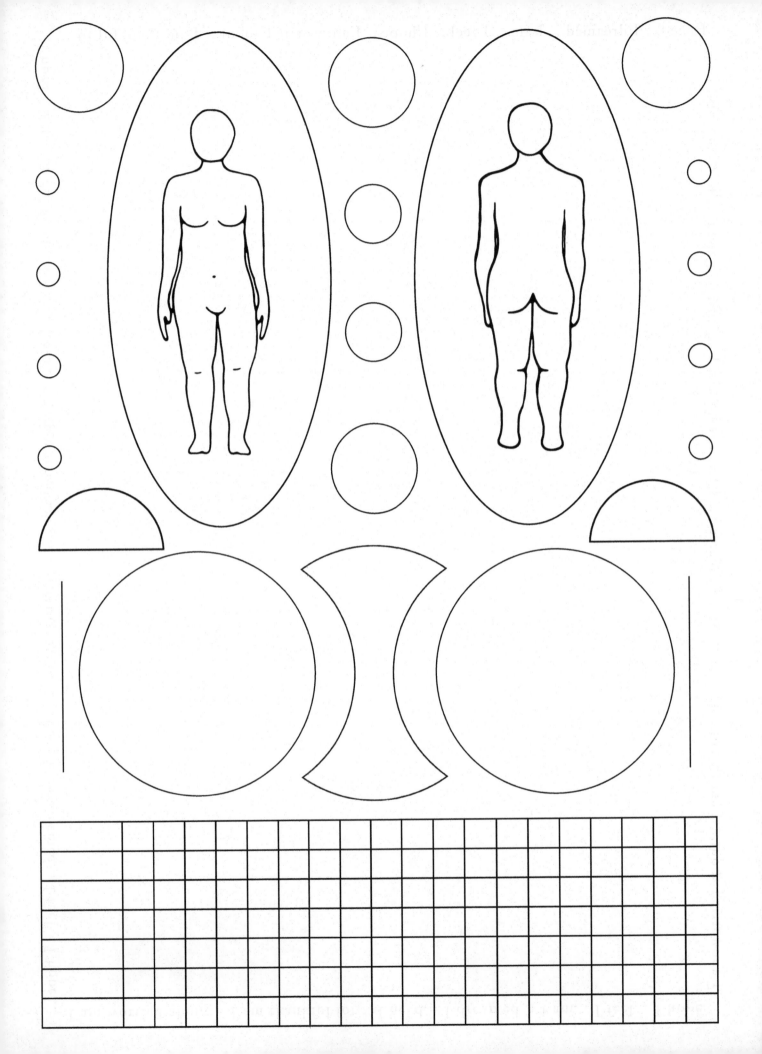

I need... I dreamed... I am... I feel... I hope... I am worried about... I am thankful for...

I need... I dreamed... I am... I feel... I hope... I am worried about... I am thankful for... I need... I dreamed... I feel... I hope...

I am worried about... I am thankful for... I need... I dreamed... I feel... I hope... I am worried about... I am thankful for... I need... I dreamed... I feel... I hope...

I am worried about... I am thankful for... I need... I dreamed... I am... I feel... I hope...

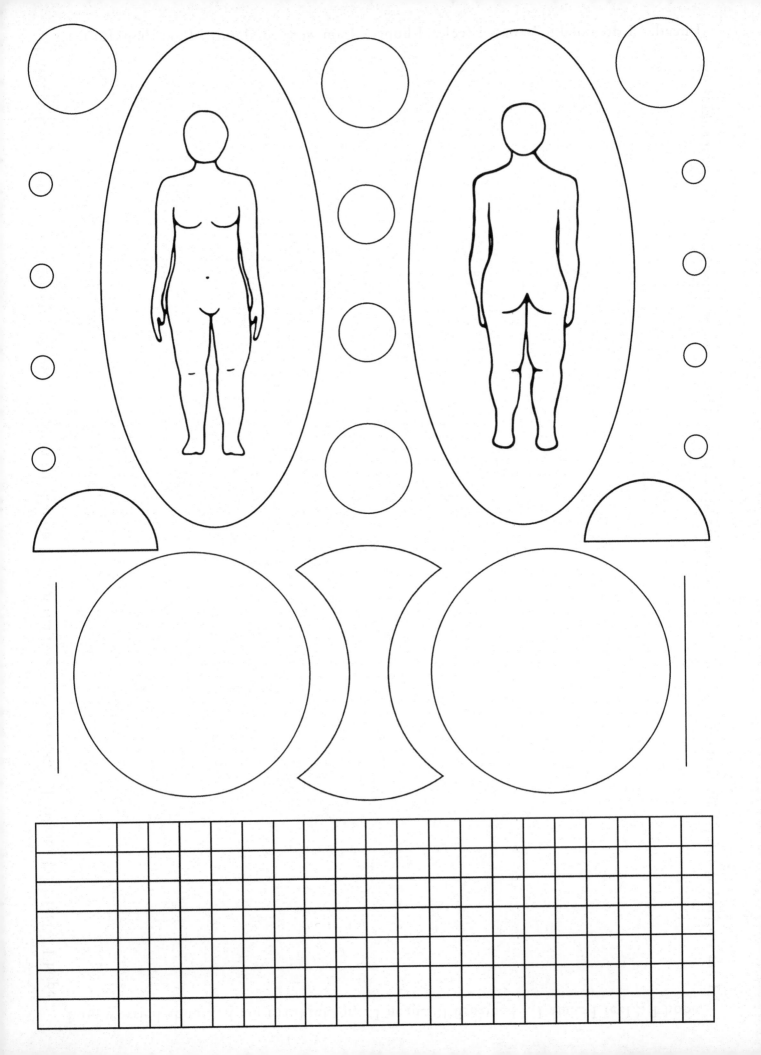

I need... I dreamed... I am... I feel... I hope... I am worried about... I am thankful for...

I need... I dreamed... I am... I feel... I hope... I am worried about... I am thankful for... I need... I dreamed... I feel... I hope...

I am worried about... I am thankful for... I need... I dreamed... I feel... I hope...

I need... I dreamed... I am... I feel... I hope... I am worried about... I am thankful for...

I am worried about... I am thankful for... I need... I dreamed... I am... I feel... I hope...

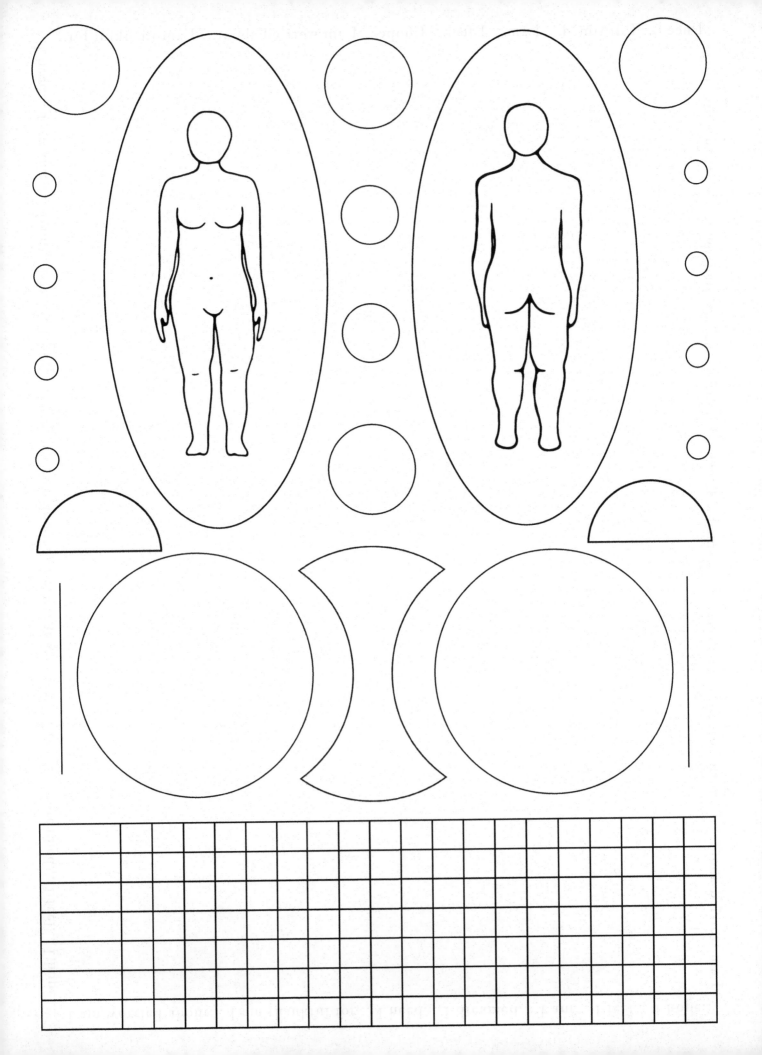

I need... I dreamed... I am... I feel... I hope... I am worried about... I am thankful for...

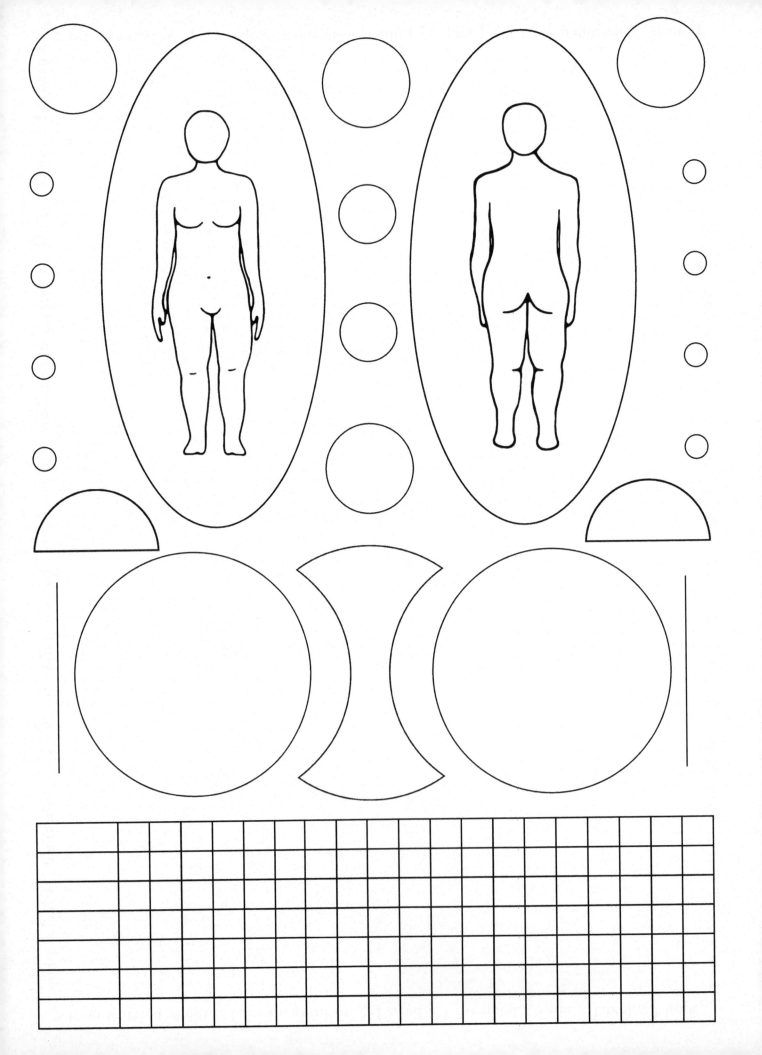

I need... I dreamed... I am... I feel... I hope... I am worried about... I am thankful for...

I need... I dreamed... I am... I feel... I hope... I am worried about... I am thankful for... I need... I dreamed... I feel... I hope...

I need... I dreamed... I feel... I hope... I am worried about... I am thankful for... I need... I dreamed... I feel... I hope... I am worried about... I am thankful for...

I am worried about... I am thankful for... I need... I dreamed... I am... I feel... I hope...

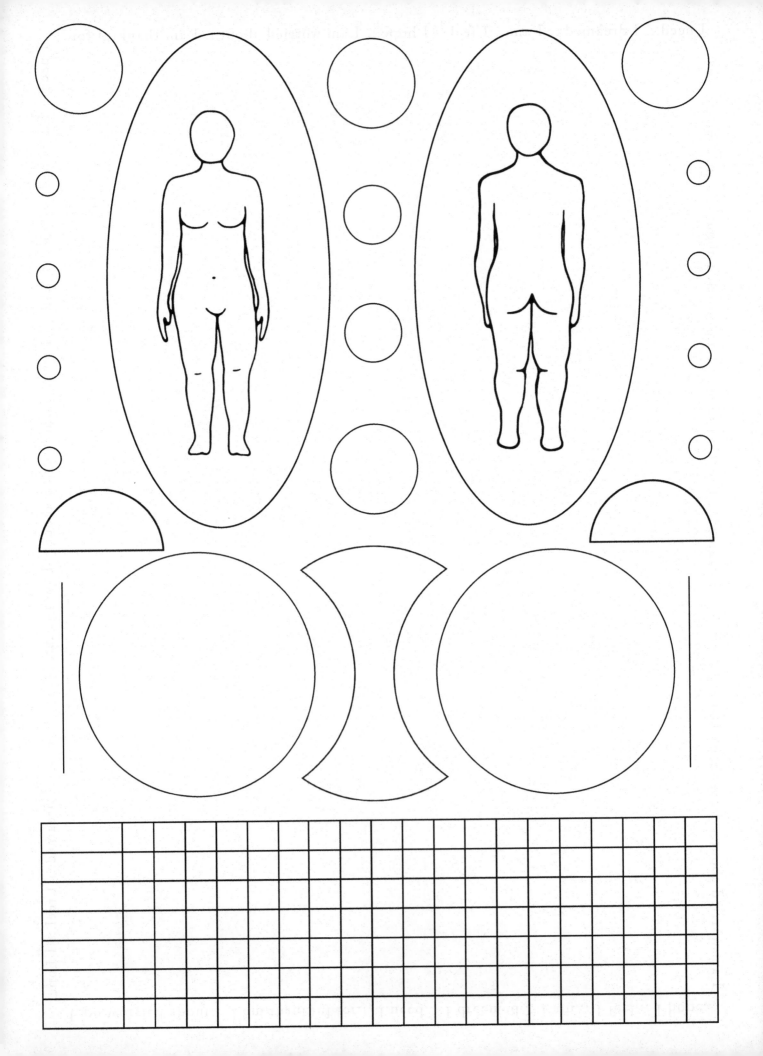

I need... I dreamed... I am... I feel... I hope... I am worried about... I am thankful for...

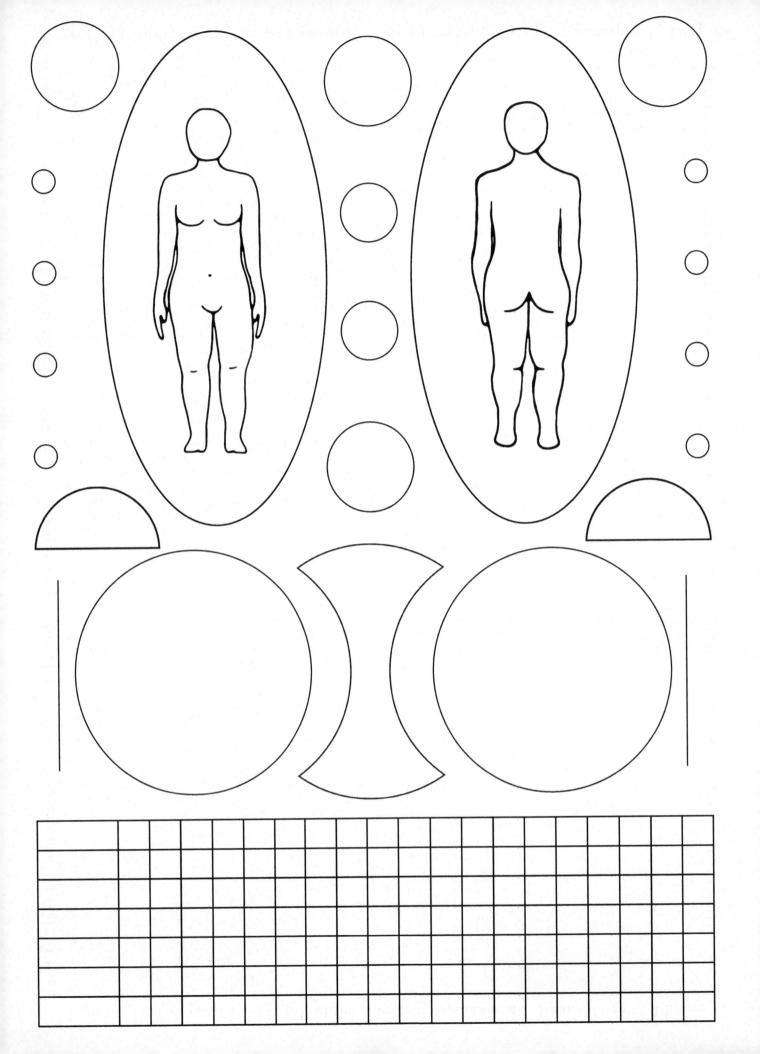

I need... I dreamed... I am... I feel... I hope... I am worried about... I am thankful for...

I need... I dreamed... I am... I feel... I hope... I am worried about... I am thankful for... I need... I dreamed... I feel... I hope...

I am thankful for... I need... I dreamed... I feel... I hope... I am worried about... I am thankful for... I need... I dreamed... I feel... I hope...

I am worried about... I am thankful for... I need... I dreamed... I feel... I am... I dreamed... I need... I am thankful for... I am worried about...

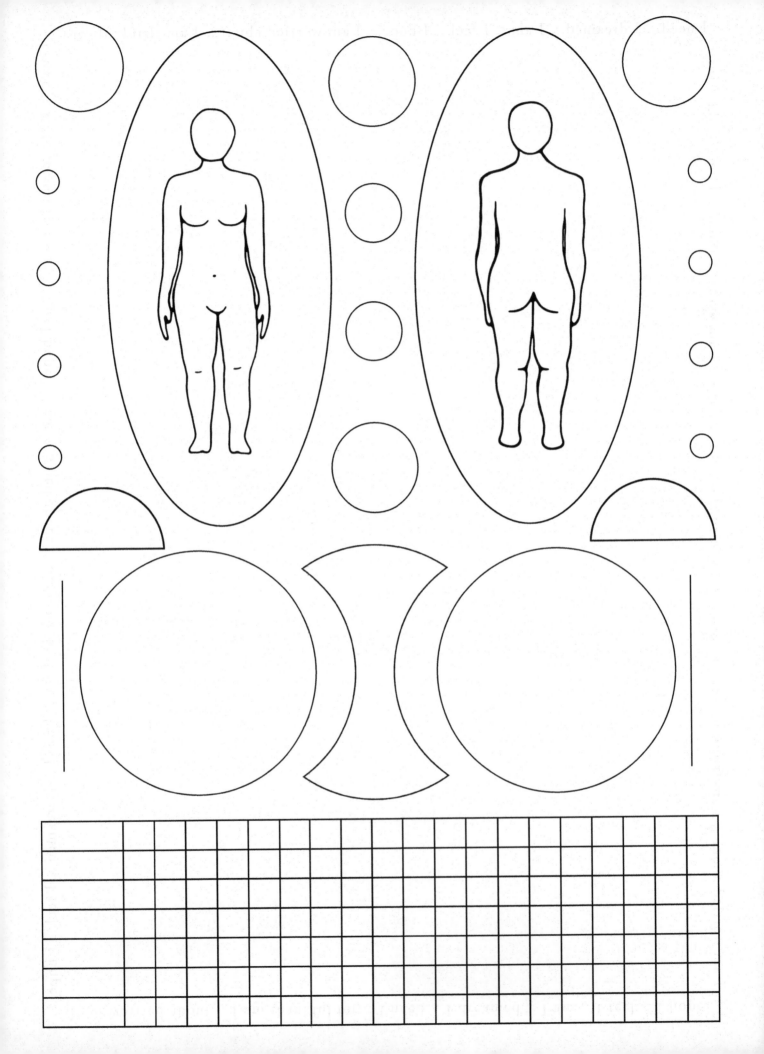

I need... I dreamed... I am... I feel... I hope... I am worried about... I am thankful for...

I need... I dreamed... I am... I feel... I hope... I am worried about... I am thankful for... I need... I dreamed... I feel... I hope...

I am worried about... I am thankful for... I need... I dreamed... I feel... I hope... I am worried about... I am thankful for...

I am worried about... I am thankful for... I need... I dreamed... I feel... I am... I hope...

I am worried about... I am thankful for... I need... I dreamed... I feel... I am... I hope...

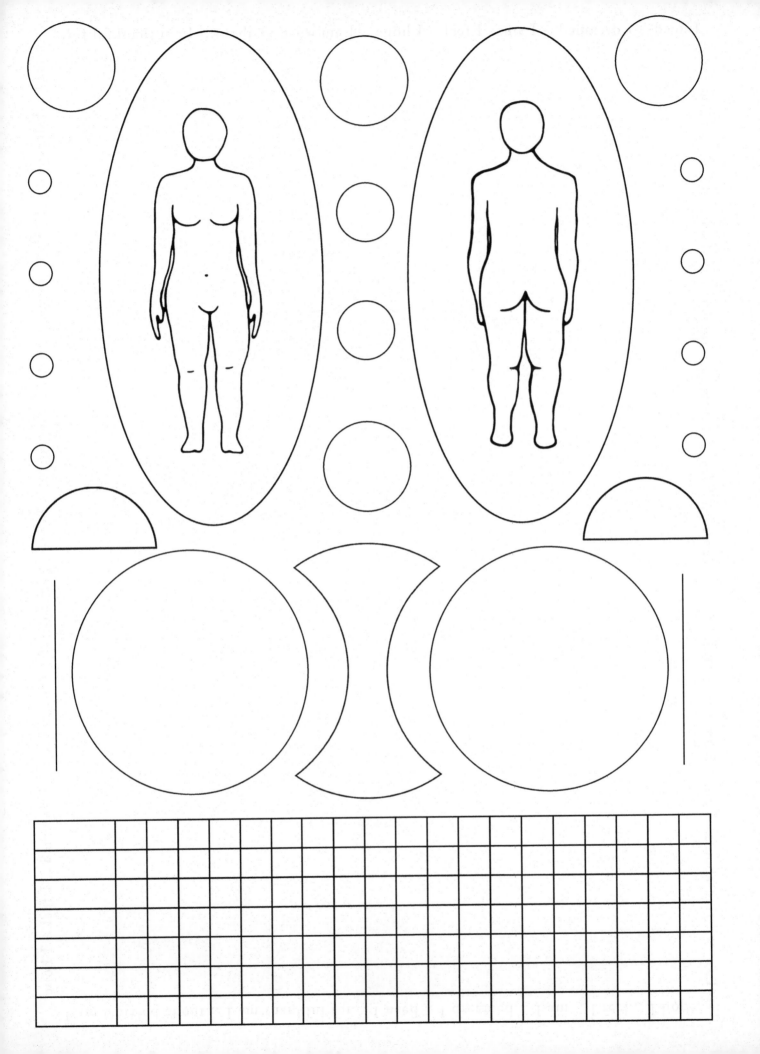

I need... I dreamed... I am... I feel... I hope... I am worried about... I am thankful for...

I need... I dreamed... I am... I feel... I hope... I am worried about... I am thankful for... I need... I dreamed... I feel... I hope...

I am thankful for... I need... I dreamed... I feel... I hope... I am worried about... I am thankful for... I am worried about...

I am worried about... I am thankful for... I need... I dreamed... I feel... I hope...

I am worried about... I am thankful for... I need... I dreamed... I am... I feel... I hope...

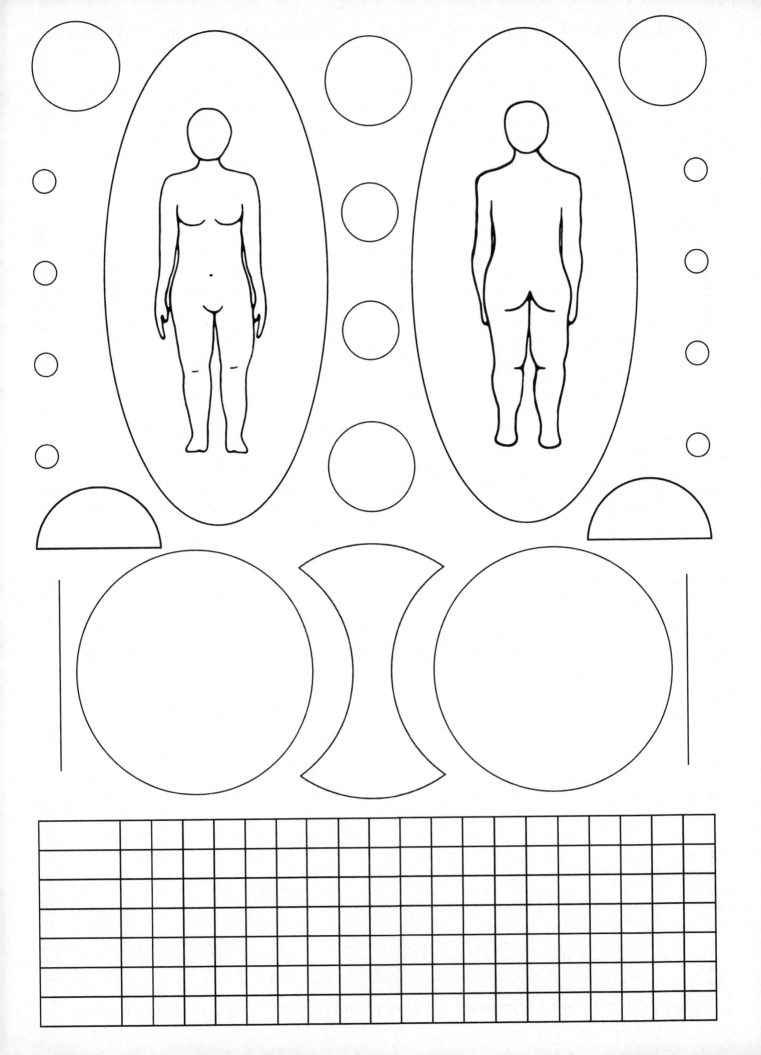

I need... I dreamed... I am... I feel... I hope... I am worried about... I am thankful for...

I need... I dreamed... I am... I feel... I hope... I am worried about... I am thankful for... I need... I dreamed... I feel... I hope...

I am thankful for... I need... I dreamed... I feel... I hope... I am worried about... I am thankful for... I need... I dreamed... I feel... I hope...

I am worried about... I am thankful for... I need... I dreamed... I am... I feel... I hope...

I am worried about... I am thankful for... I need... I dreamed... I am... I feel... I hope...

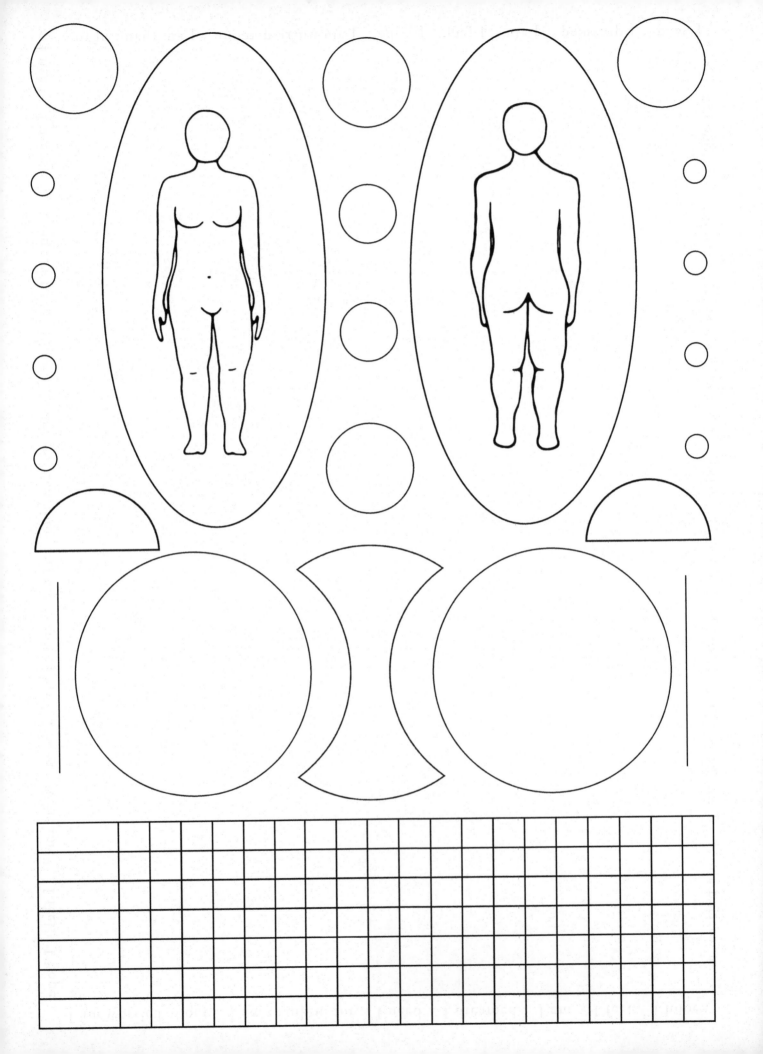

I need... I dreamed... I am... I feel... I hope... I am worried about... I am thankful for...

I need... I dreamed... I am... I feel... I hope... I am worried about... I am thankful for... I need... I dreamed... I feel... I hope...

I am worried about... I am thankful for... I need... I dreamed... I feel... I hope... I am worried about... I am thankful for... I need... I dreamed... I feel... I hope...

I am worried about... I am thankful for... I need... I dreamed... I feel... I am... I dreamed... I need... I am thankful for... I am worried about... I hope...

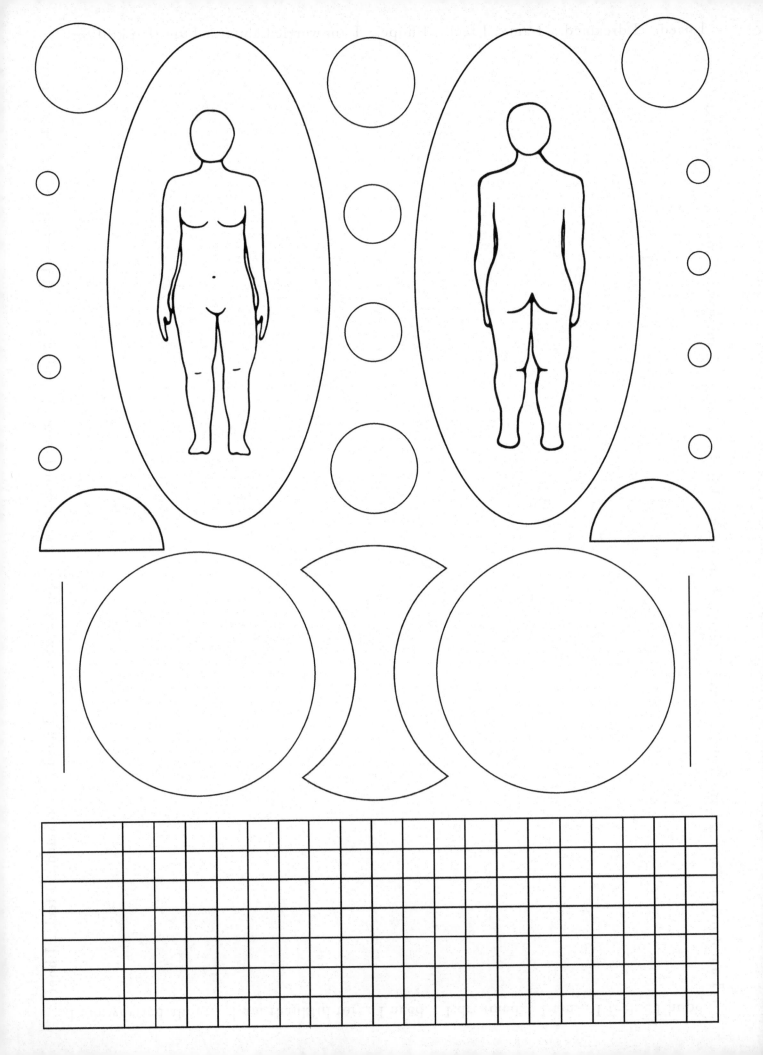

I need... I dreamed... I am... I feel... I hope... I am worried about... I am thankful for...

I need... I dreamed... I am... I feel... I hope... I am worried about... I am thankful for... I need... I dreamed... I feel... I hope...

I am thankful for... I need... I dreamed... I feel... I hope... I am worried about... I am thankful for... I need... I dreamed... I am... I feel... I hope...

I am worried about... I am thankful for... I need... I dreamed... I am... I feel... I hope...

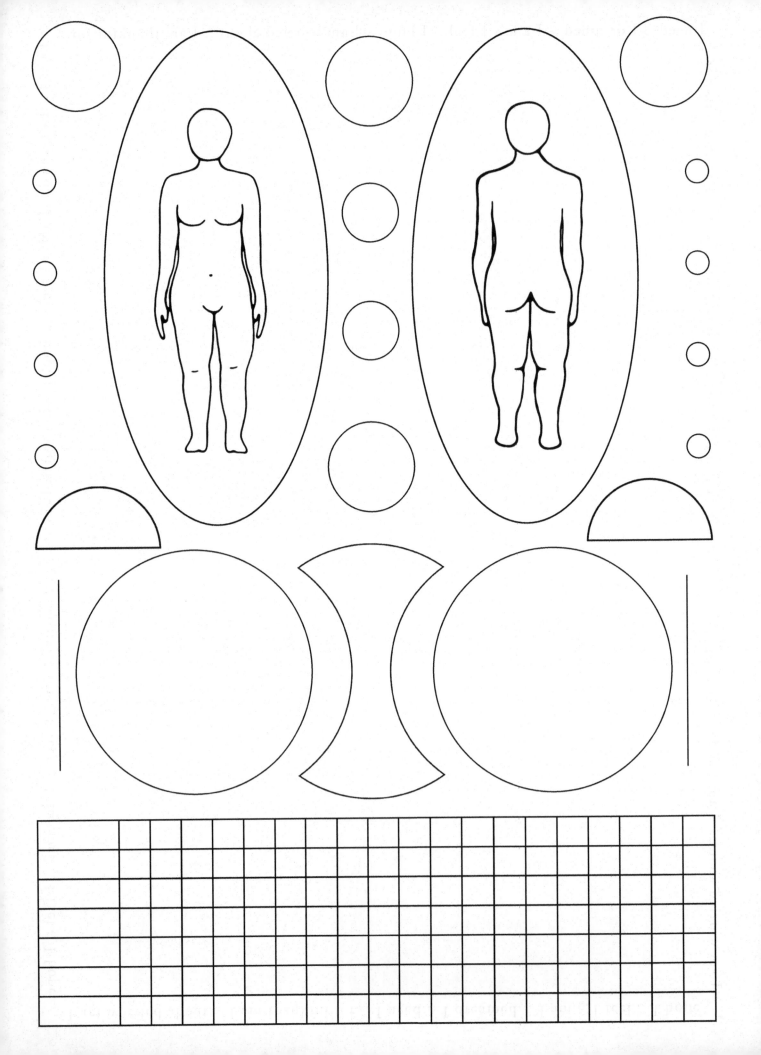

I need... I dreamed... I am... I feel... I hope... I am worried about... I am thankful for...

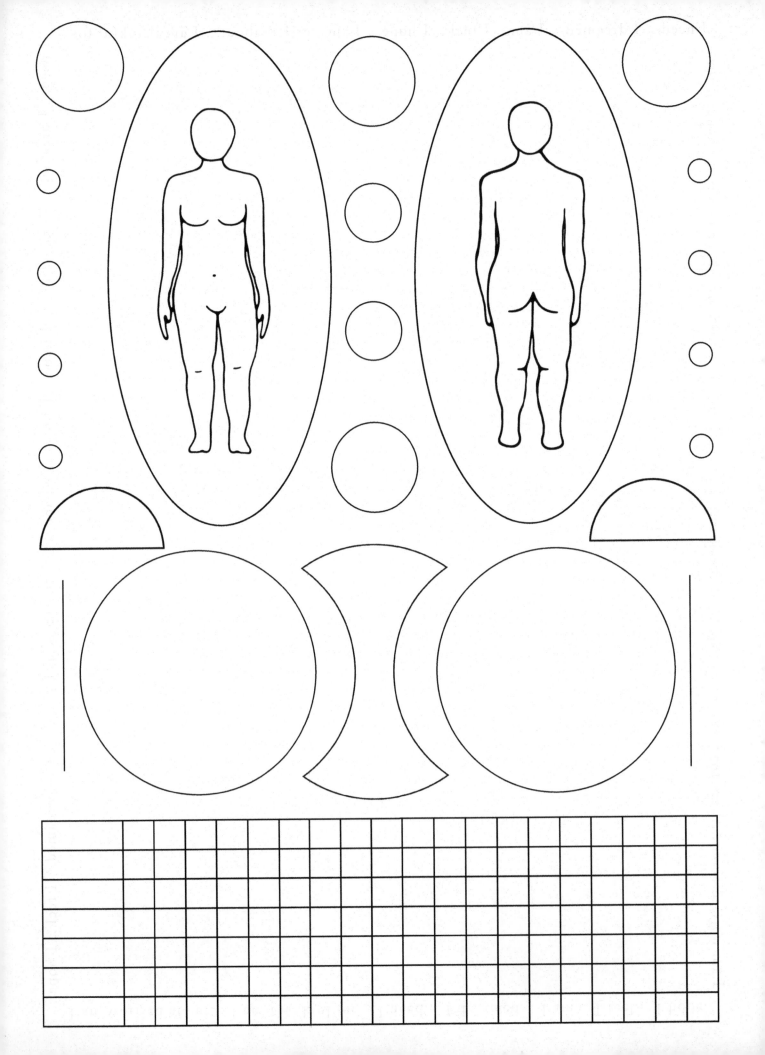

I need... I dreamed... I am... I feel... I hope... I am worried about... I am thankful for...

I need... I dreamed... I am... I feel... I hope... I am worried about... I am thankful for...

I am thankful for... I need... I dreamed... I feel... I hope... I am worried about...

I am worried about... I am thankful for... I need... I dreamed... I feel... I hope...

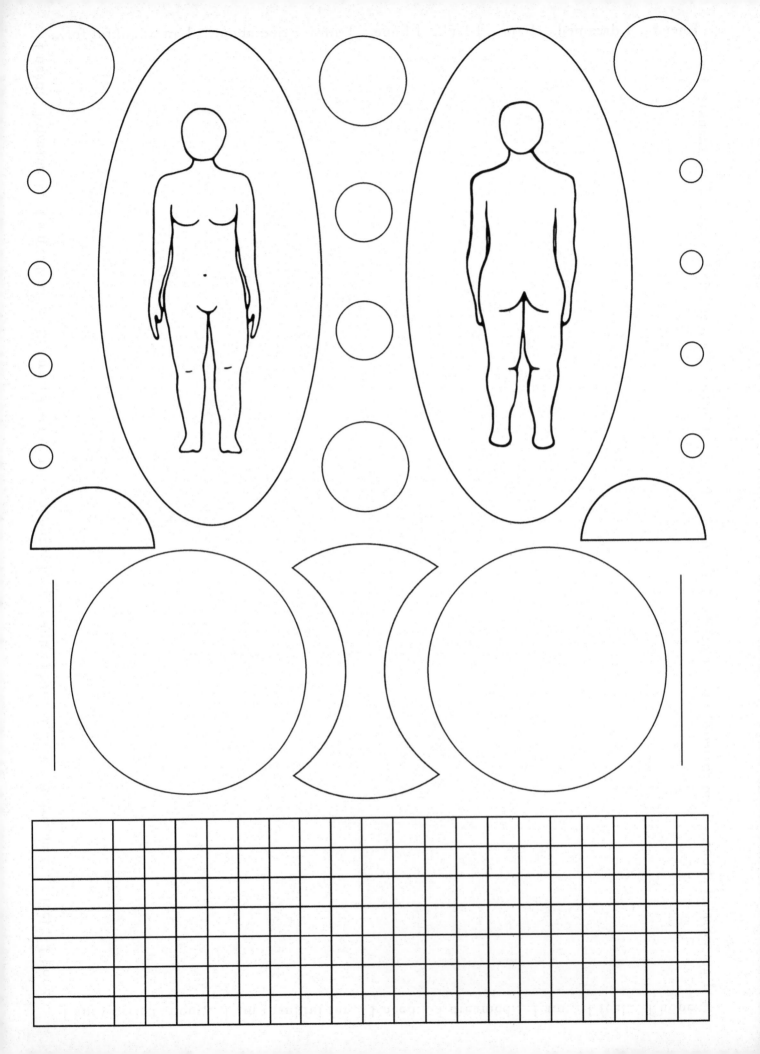

I need... I dreamed... I am... I feel... I hope... I am worried about... I am thankful for...

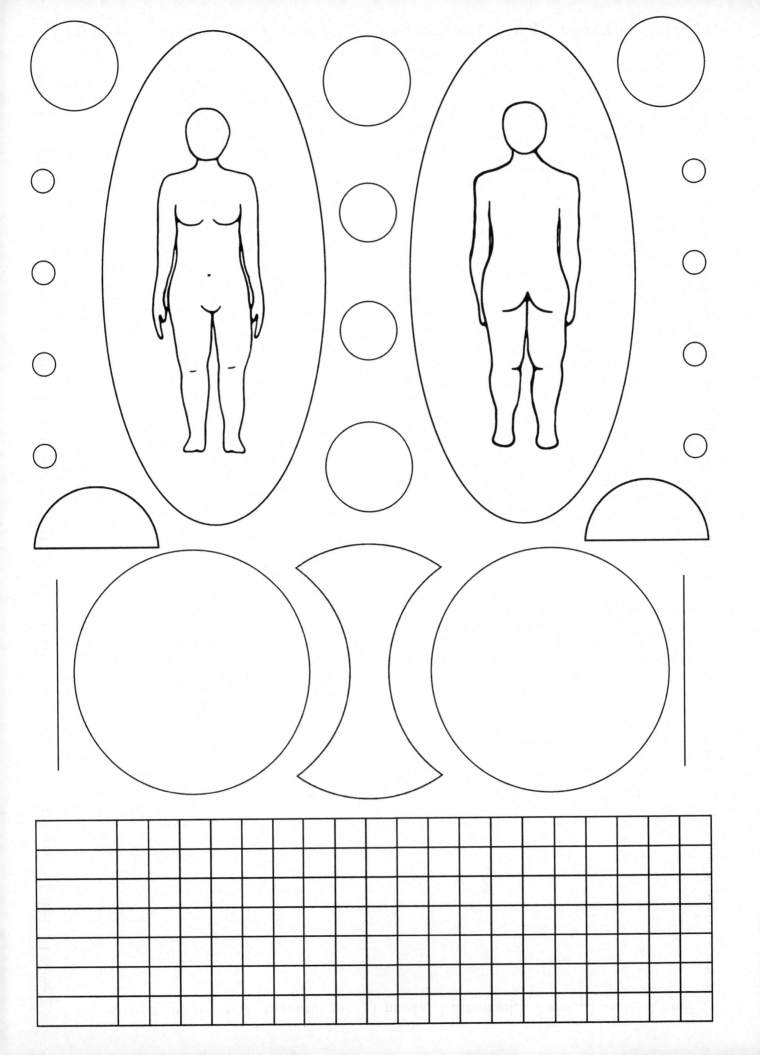

I need... I dreamed... I am... I feel... I hope... I am worried about... I am thankful for...

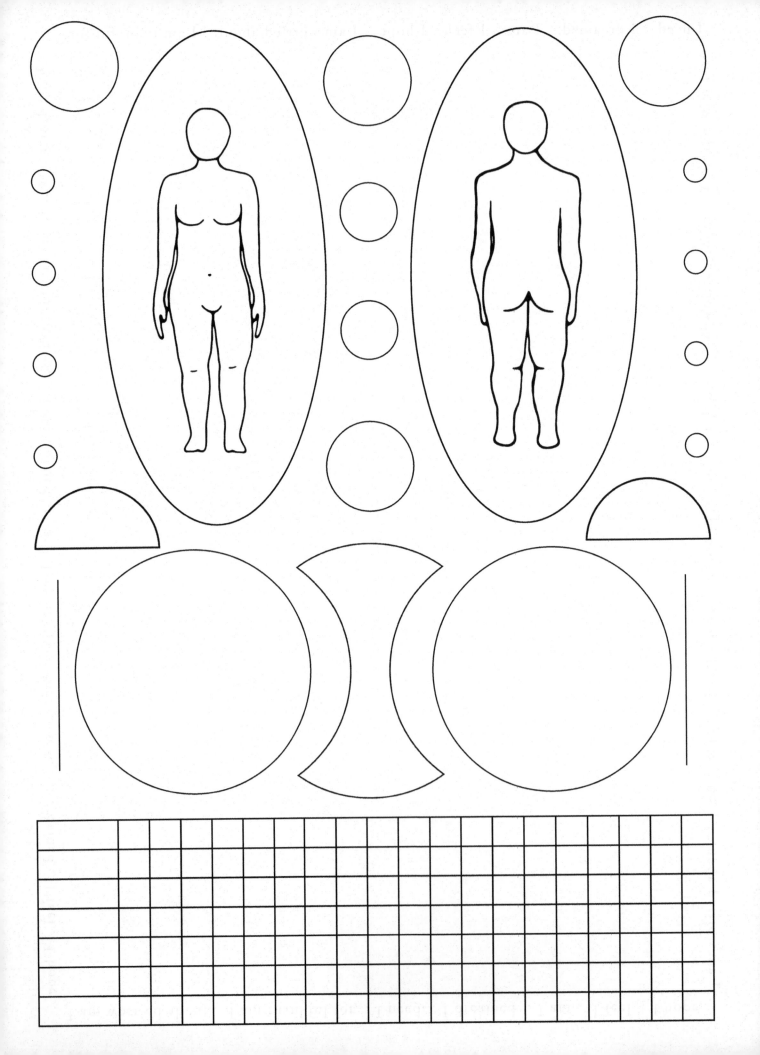

I need... I dreamed... I am... I feel... I hope... I am worried about... I am thankful for...

I need... I dreamed... I am... I feel... I hope... I am worried about... I am thankful for... I need... I dreamed... I feel... I hope...

I am worried about... I am thankful for... I need... I dreamed... I feel... I hope... I am worried about... I am thankful for... I need... I dreamed... I feel... I hope...

I am worried about... I am thankful for... I need... I dreamed... I feel... I am... I feel... I hope...

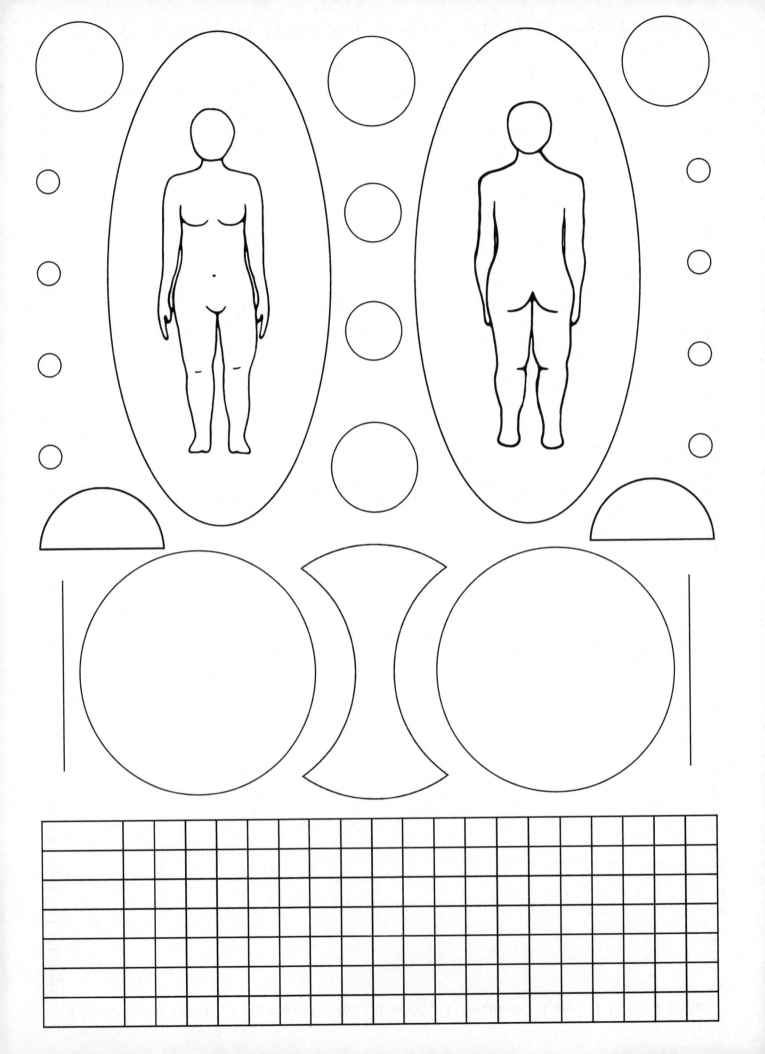

I need... I dreamed... I am... I feel... I hope... I am worried about... I am thankful for...

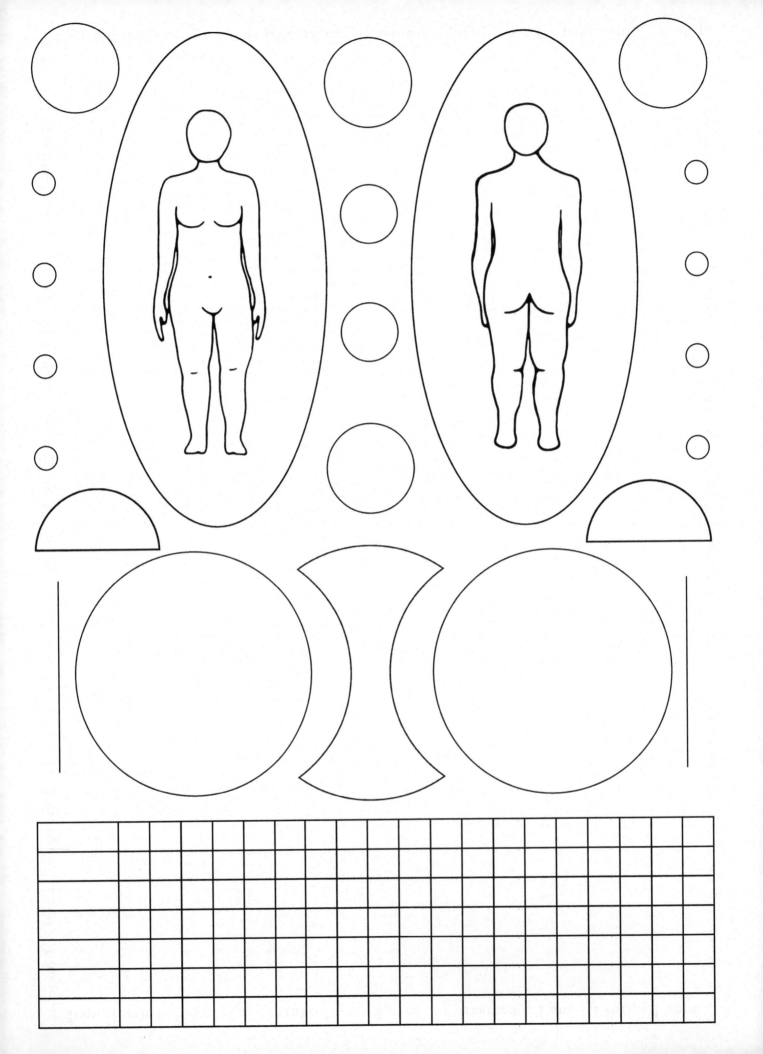

I need... I dreamed... I am... I feel... I hope... I am worried about... I am thankful for...

I need... I dreamed... I am... I feel... I hope... I am worried about... I am thankful for... I need... I dreamed... I feel... I hope...

I am worried about... I am thankful for... I need... I dreamed... I feel... I hope... I am worried about... I am thankful for...

I am worried about... I am thankful for... I need... I dreamed... I feel... I am... I hope...

I am worried about... I am thankful for... I need... I dreamed... I feel... I am... I hope...

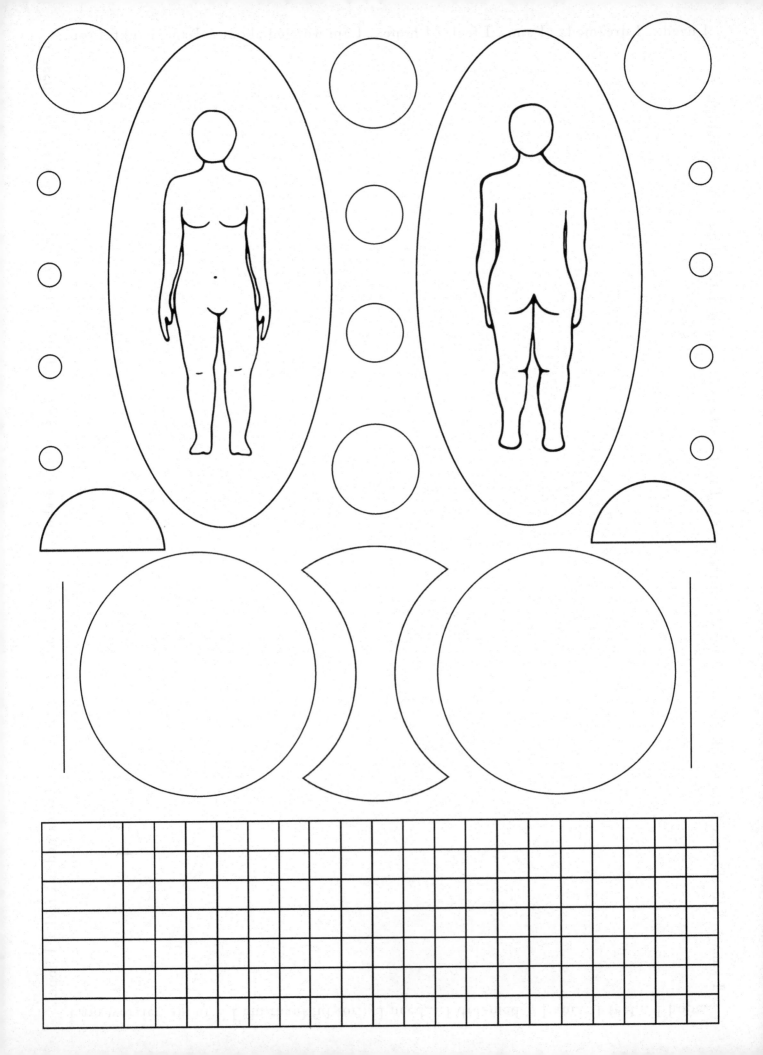

I need... I dreamed... I am... I feel... I hope... I am worried about... I am thankful for...

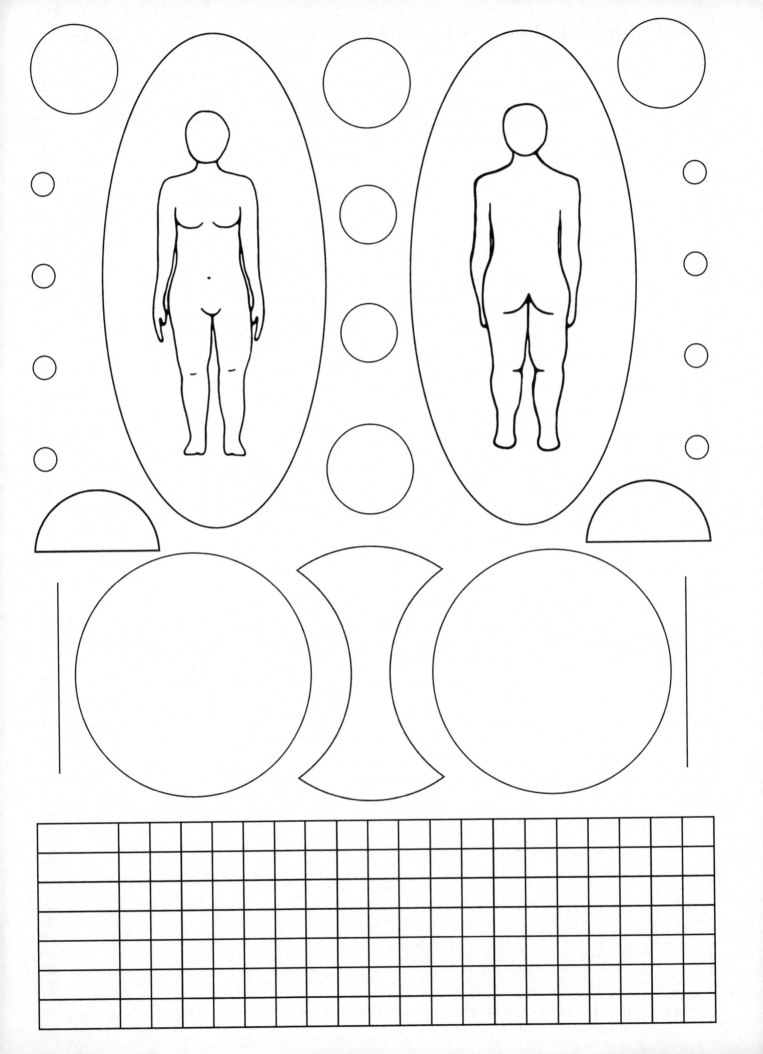

I need... I dreamed... I am... I feel... I hope... I am worried about... I am thankful for...

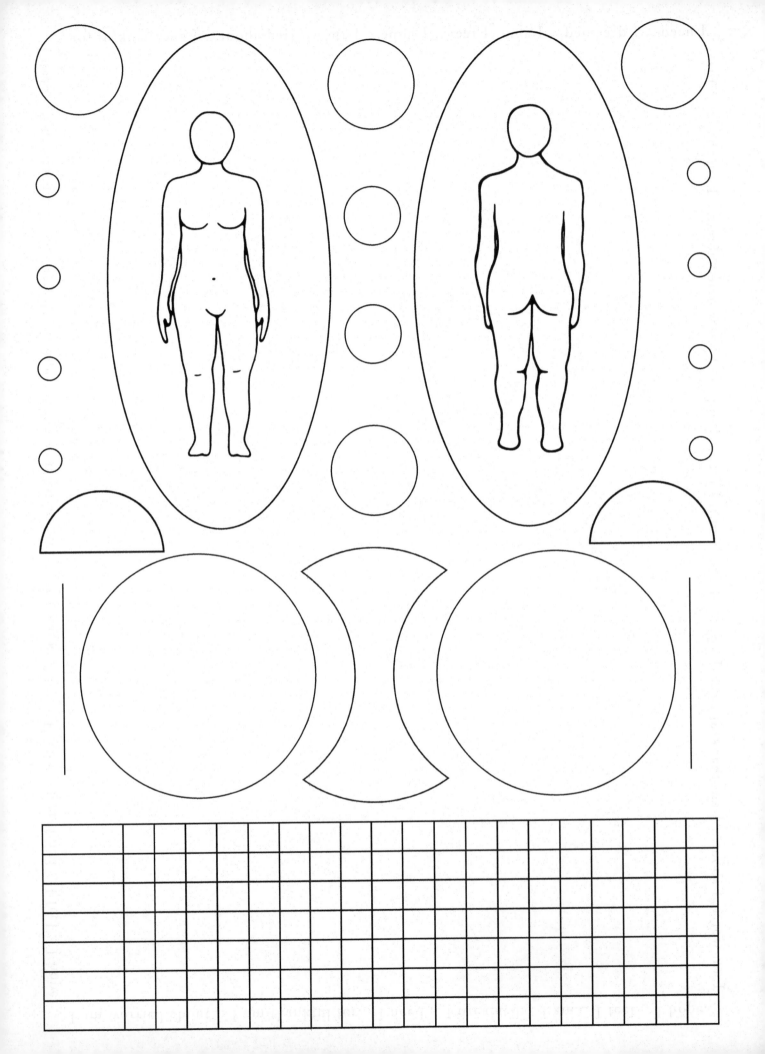

I need... I dreamed... I am... I feel... I hope... I am worried about... I am thankful for...

I need... I dreamed... I am... I feel... I hope... I am worried about... I am thankful for... I need... I dreamed... I feel... I hope...

I am worried about... I am thankful for... I need... I dreamed... I feel... I hope... I am worried about... I am thankful for... I need...

I am worried about... I am thankful for... I need... I dreamed... I am... I feel... I am worried about... I am thankful for... I hope...

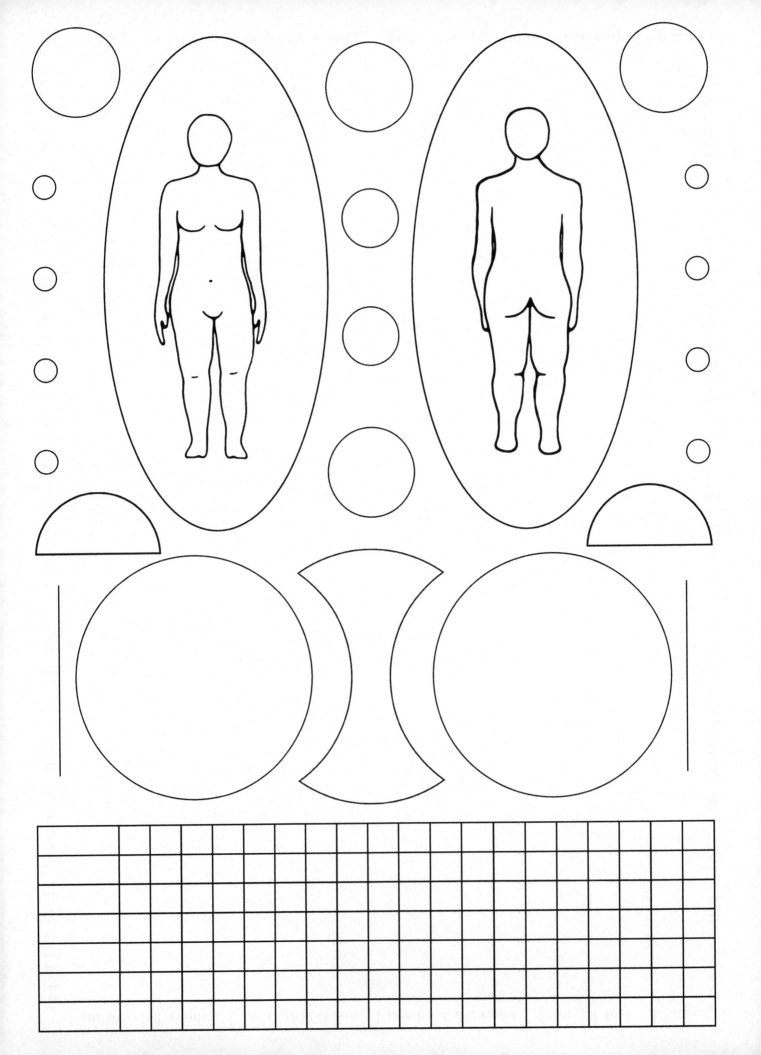

I need... I dreamed... I am... I feel... I hope... I am worried about... I am thankful for...

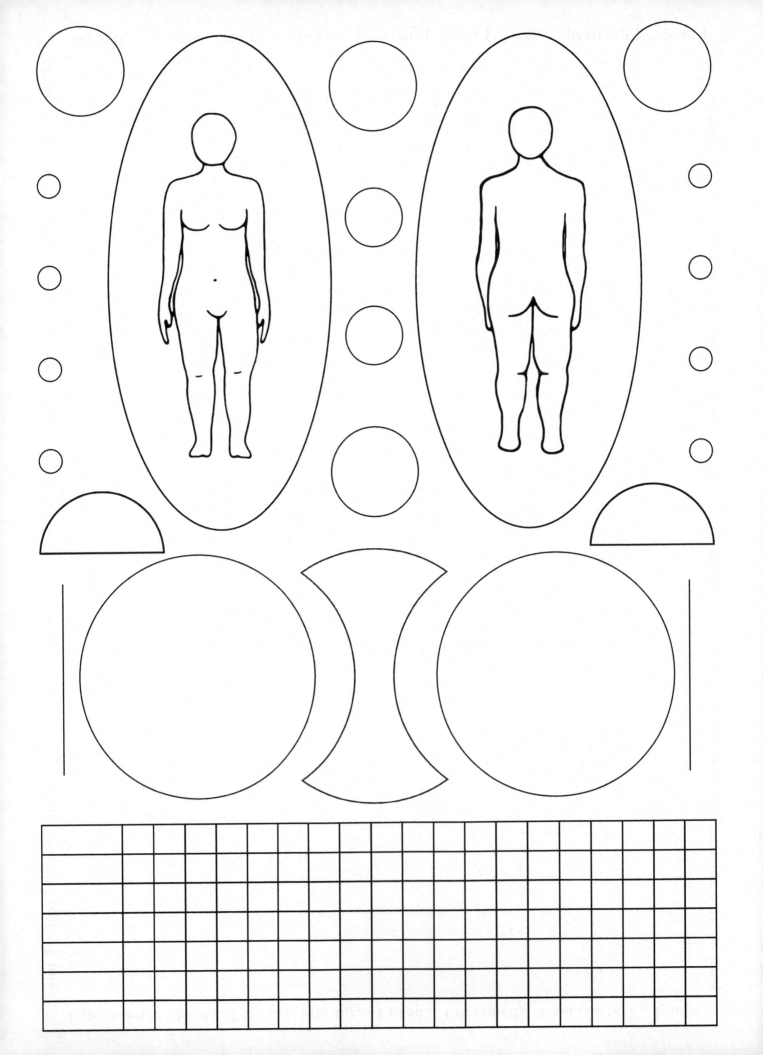

I need... I dreamed... I am... I feel... I hope... I am worried about... I am thankful for...

I need... I dreamed... I am... I feel... I hope... I am worried about... I am thankful for... I need... I dreamed... I feel... I hope...

I am worried about... I am thankful for... I need... I dreamed... I feel... I hope... I am worried about... I am thankful for... I need...

I am worried about... I am thankful for... I need... I dreamed... I feel... I am... I dreamed... I need... I feel... I hope...

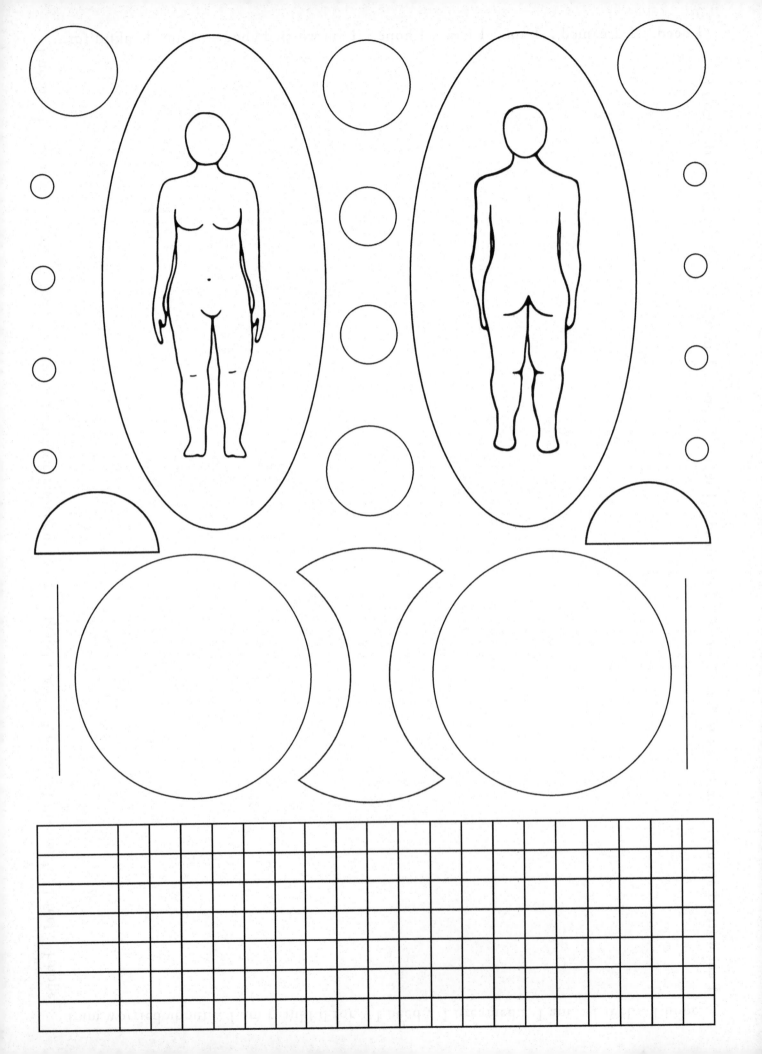

I need... I dreamed... I am... I feel... I hope... I am worried about... I am thankful for...

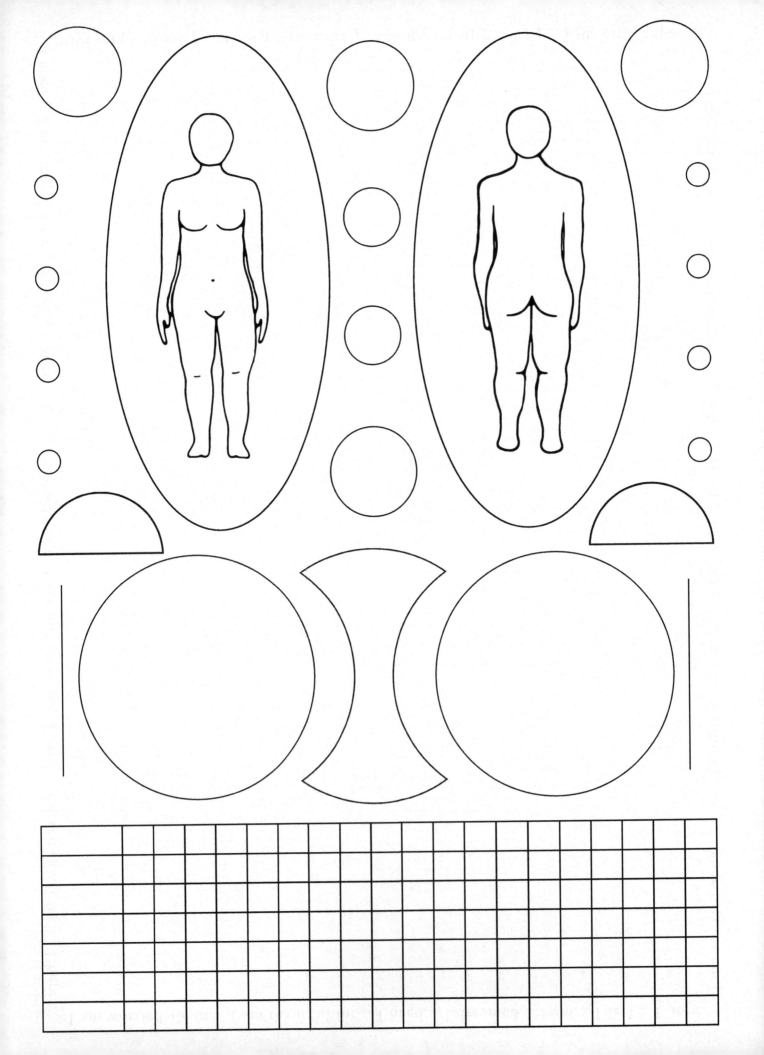

I need... I dreamed... I am... I feel... I hope... I am worried about... I am thankful for...

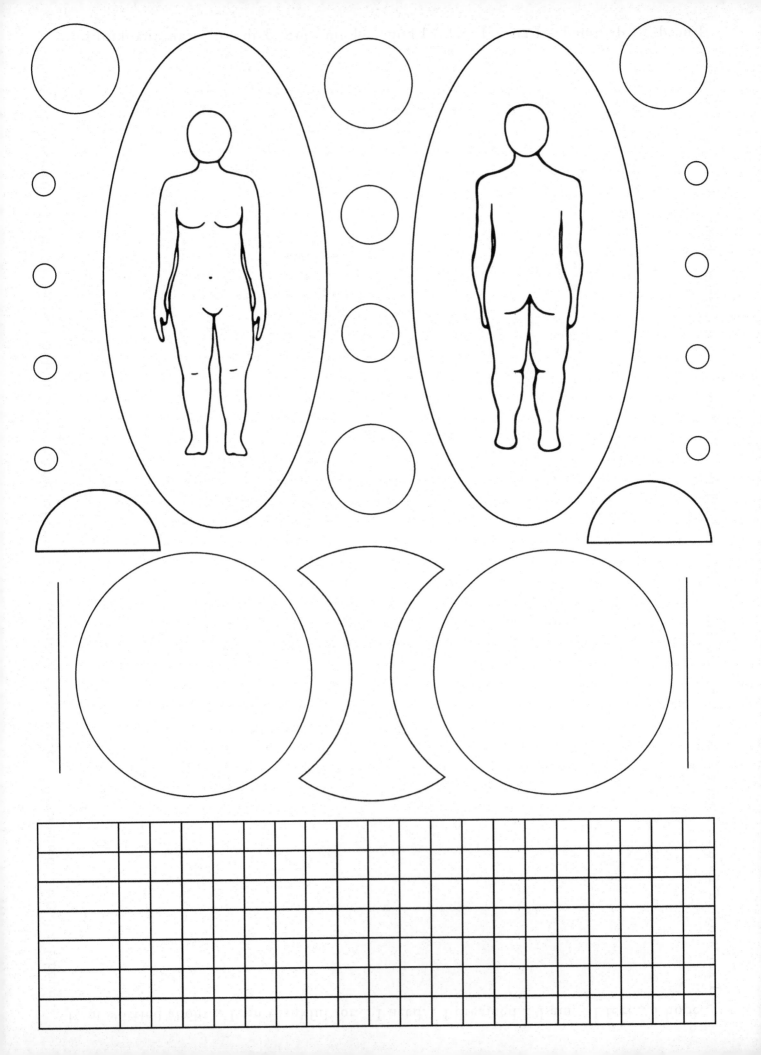

I need... I dreamed... I am... I feel... I hope... I am worried about... I am thankful for...

I need... I dreamed... I am... I feel... I hope... I am worried about... I am thankful for... I need... I dreamed... I feel... I hope...

I am thankful for... I need... I dreamed... I feel... I hope... I am worried about... I am thankful for...

I am worried about... I am thankful for... I need... I dreamed... I feel... I am... I hope...

I am worried about... I am thankful for... I need... I dreamed... I feel... I am... I hope...

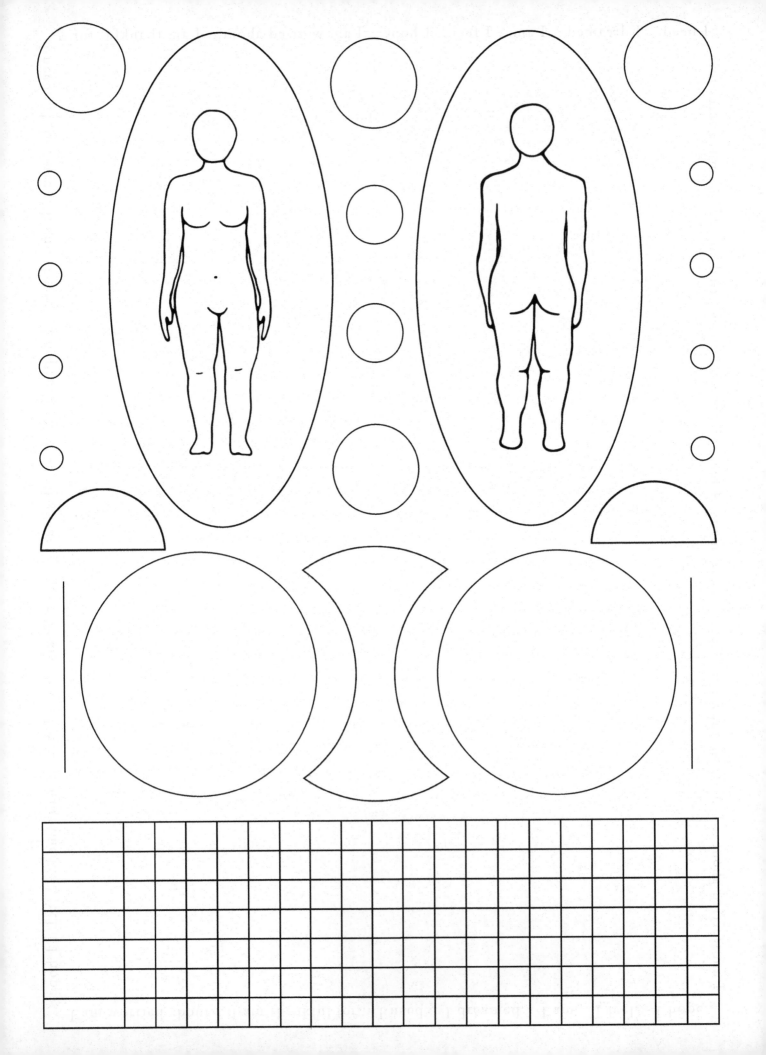

I need... I dreamed... I am... I feel... I hope... I am worried about... I am thankful for...

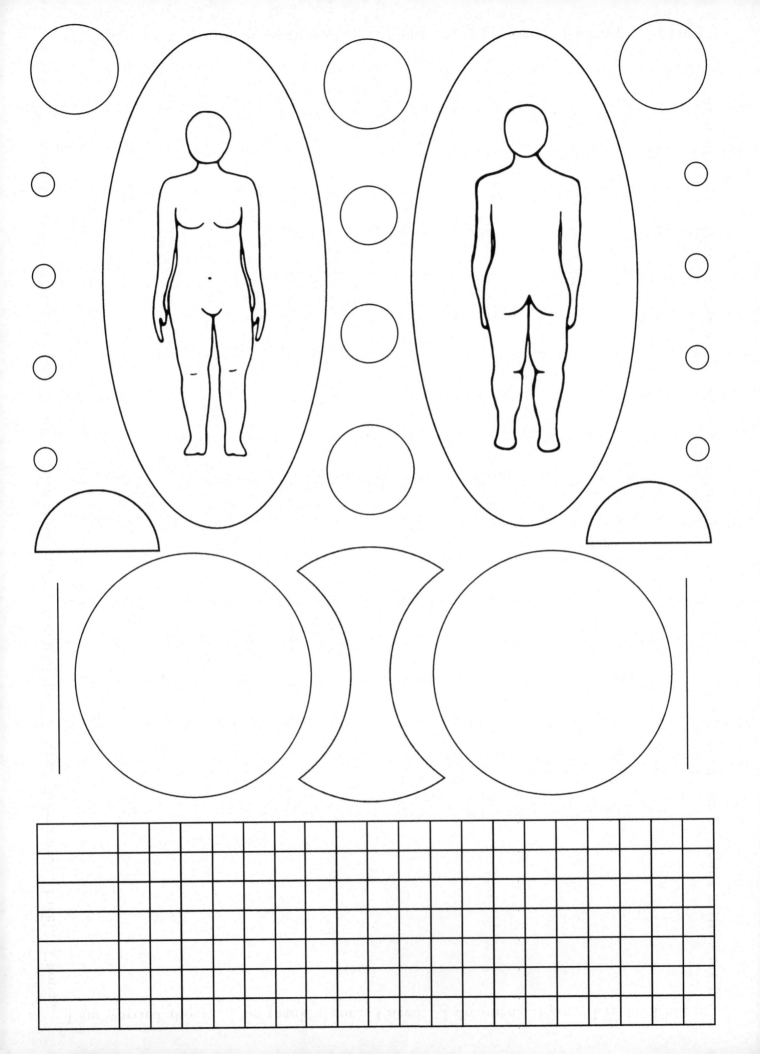

I need... I dreamed... I am... I feel... I hope... I am worried about... I am thankful for...

I need... I dreamed... I am... I feel... I hope... I am worried about... I am thankful for... I need... I dreamed... I feel... I hope...

I am thankful for... I need... I dreamed... I feel... I hope... I am worried about... I am thankful for... I need... I dreamed... I feel... I hope... I am worried about...

I am worried about... I am thankful for... I need... I dreamed... I feel... I am... I dreamed... I need... I am thankful for... I am worried about... I hope...

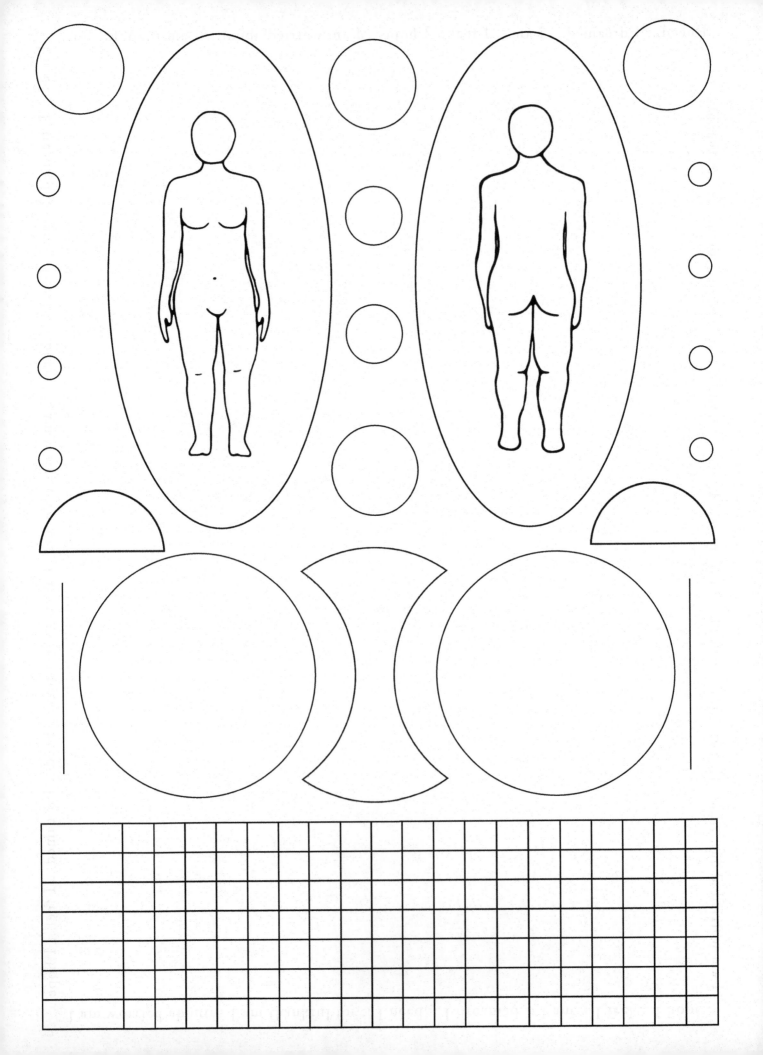

I need... I dreamed... I am... I feel... I hope... I am worried about... I am thankful for...

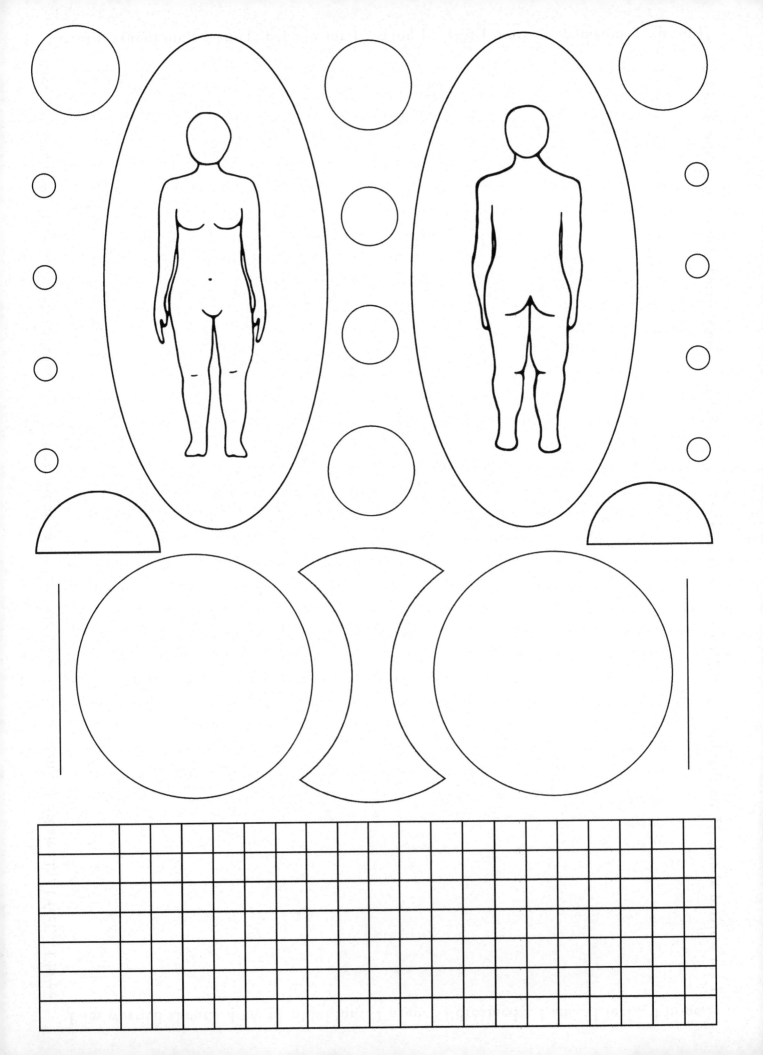

I need... I dreamed... I am... I feel... I hope... I am worried about... I am thankful for...

I need... I dreamed... I am... I feel... I hope... I am worried about... I am thankful for... I need... I dreamed... I feel... I hope...

I am thankful for... I need... I dreamed... I feel... I hope... I am worried about... I am thankful for... I need... I dreamed... I feel... I hope...

I am worried about... I am thankful for... I need... I dreamed... I feel... I am... I hope...

I am worried about... I am thankful for... I need... I dreamed... I feel... I am... I hope...

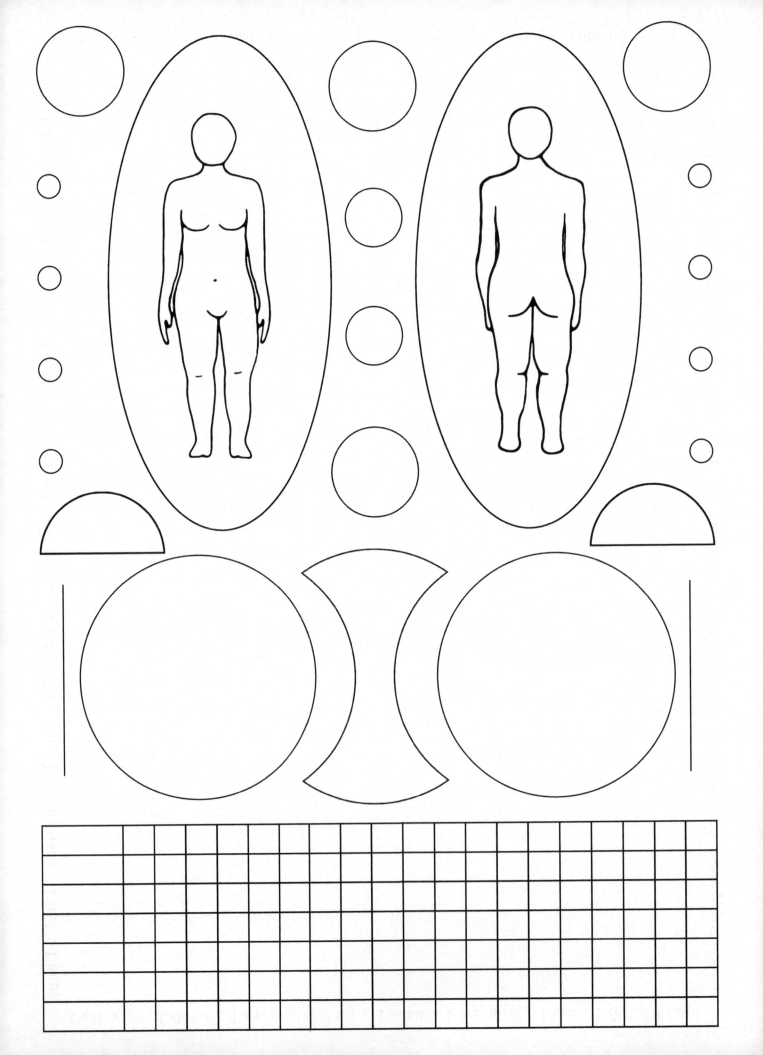

I need... I dreamed... I am... I feel... I hope... I am worried about... I am thankful for...

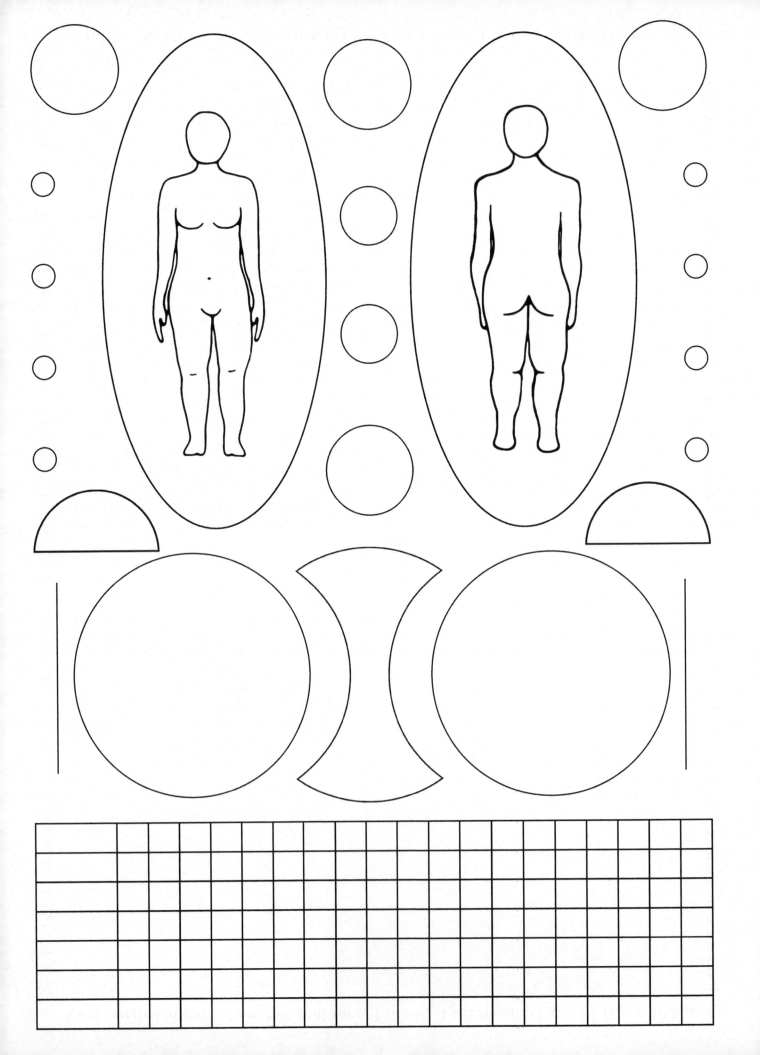

I need... I dreamed... I am... I feel... I hope... I am worried about... I am thankful for...

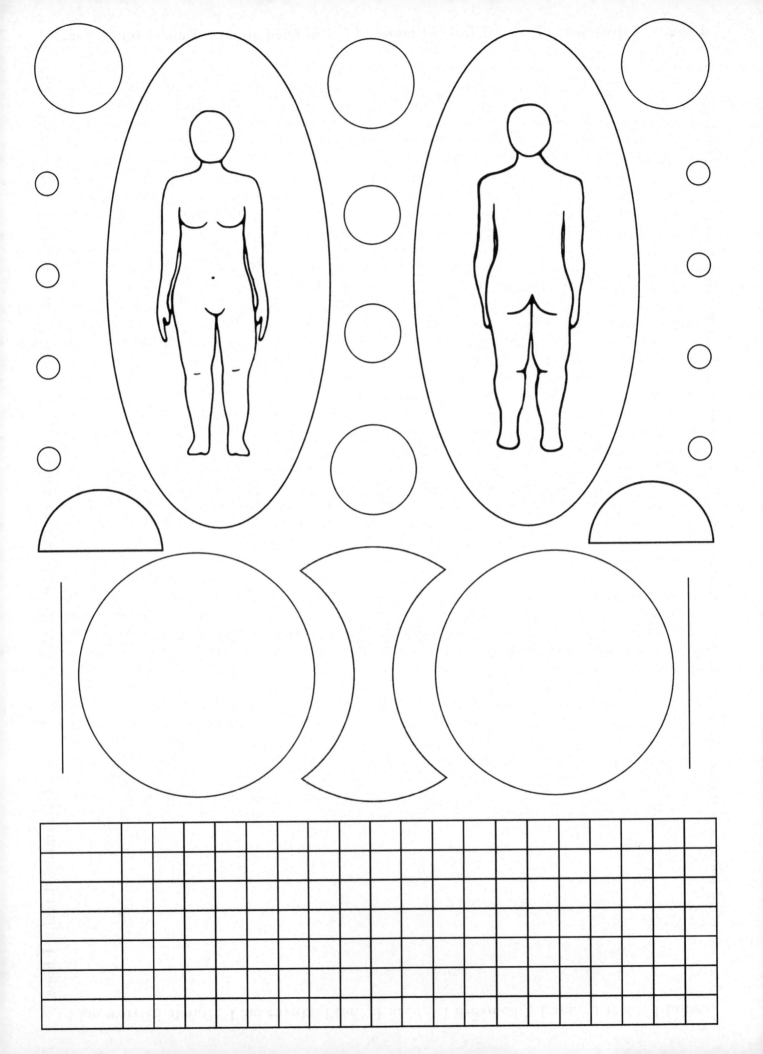

I need... I dreamed... I am... I feel... I hope... I am worried about... I am thankful for...

I need... I dreamed... I am... I feel... I hope... I am worried about... I am thankful for... I need... I dreamed... I feel... I hope...

I am thankful for... I need... I dreamed... I feel... I hope... I am worried about... I am thankful for... I need... I dreamed... I feel... I hope... I am worried about... I am thankful for... I need...

I am worried about... I am thankful for... I need... I dreamed... I feel... I am... I dreamed... I need... I need... I am thankful for... I am worried about... I am worried about... I hope...

I am worried about... I am thankful for... I need... I dreamed... I feel... I am... I am thankful for... I need... I dreamed... I feel... I hope...

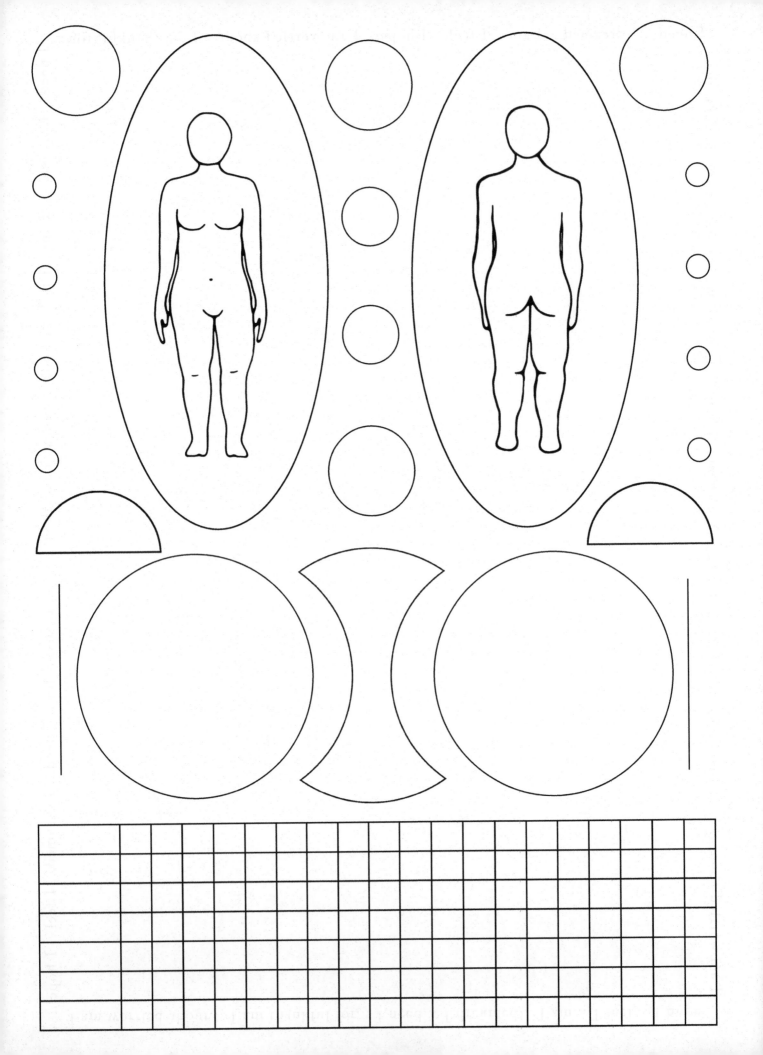

I need... I dreamed... I am... I feel... I hope... I am worried about... I am thankful for...

My
Monthly Review
Pages

MONTH:

Take a look at all your information in the Monthly Tracker and reflect:

What patterns do you notice? What things cluster together? Does anything surprise you?

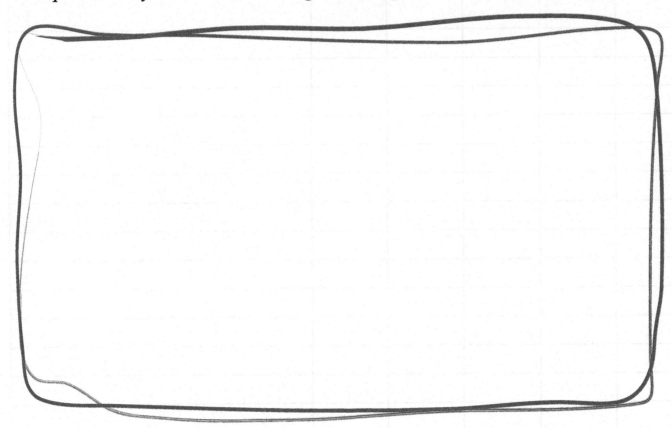

Look at the days preceding any ill health – do you see any patterns, triggers or clues?

Which combination of events seem to signal good health or illness?

How do the days of your menstrual cycle relate to: health, exercise, energy, spirtuality, mood, creativity and libido?

Goals Set | Achievements

Pressure Points	Power Points

This month's illnesses

Illness	Duration	Triggers / Causes

How I healed | What it represents on a symbolic level

What's happening in your circles this month?

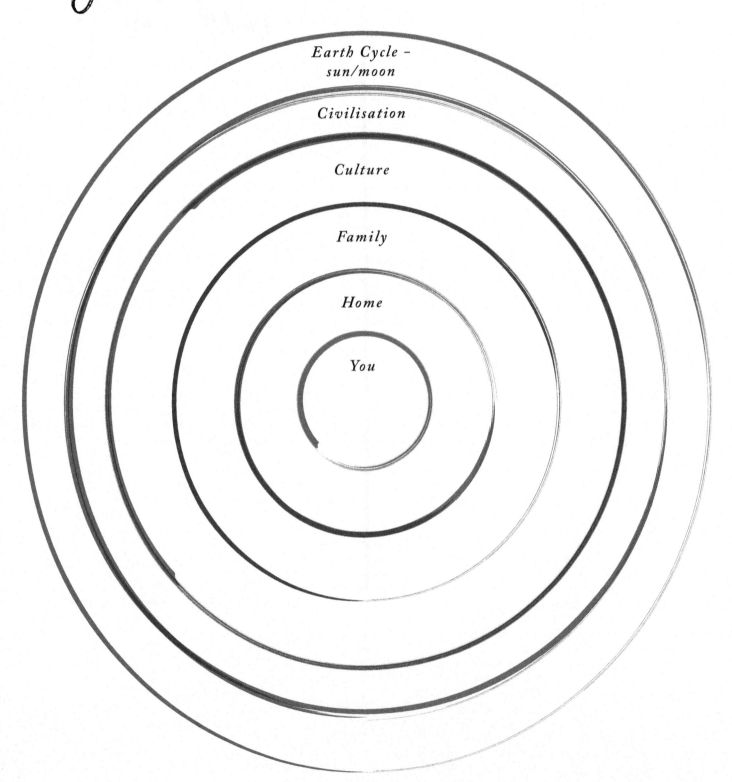

Earth Cycle –
sun/moon

Civilisation

Culture

Family

Home

You

This Month's Cycle Circles

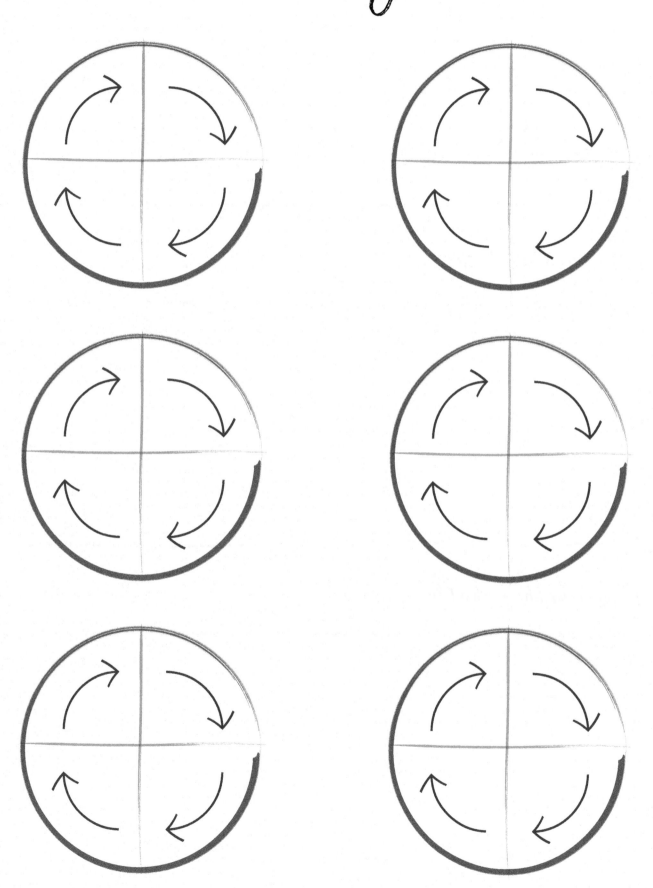

This month I am proud that...

I am grateful for...

This month's challenges were...

My health concerns this month...

- ○
- ○
- ○
- ○

I will address these by...

- ○
- ○
- ○
- ○

Appointments I need to make for next month:

- ○ Therapist/Counsellor
- ○ Doctor
- ○ Dentist/Dental hygienist
- ○ Hospital
- ○ Chiropractor/Osteopath
- ○ Physiotherapist

- ○ Massage
- ○ Smear/Mammogram
- ○ ....
- ○ ....
- ○ ....
- ○ ....

Full Circle Chart
(30 days)

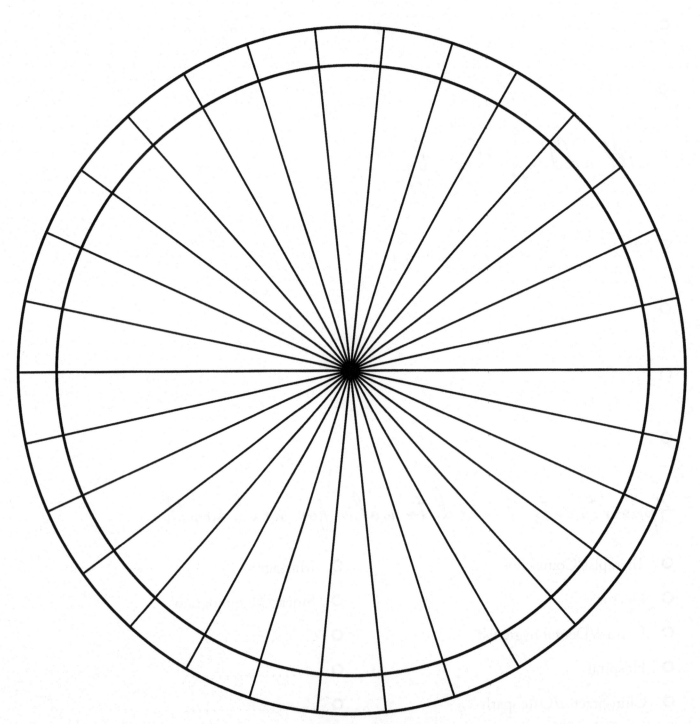

Full Circle Chart

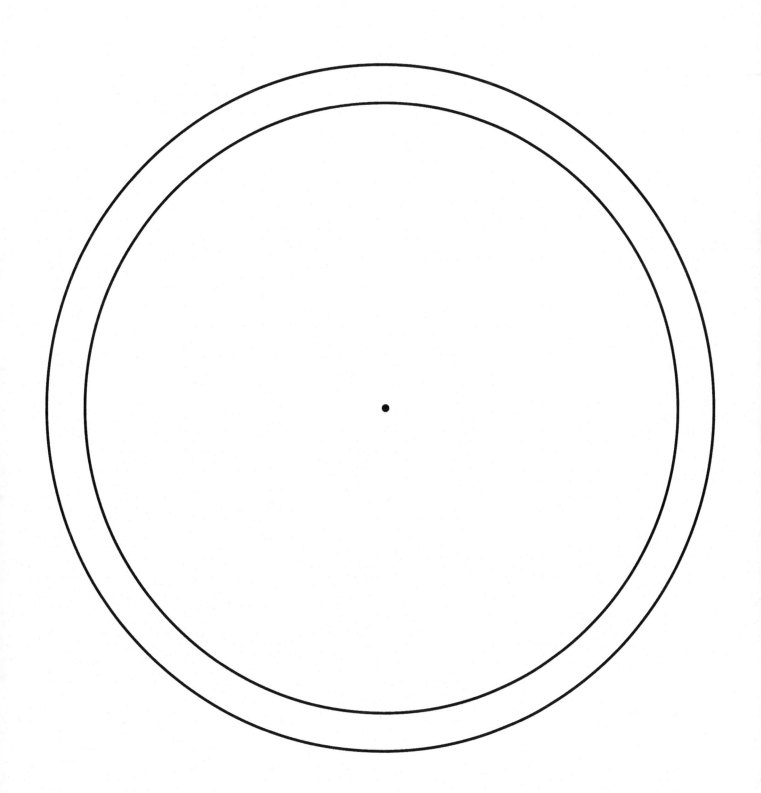

About the author

LUCY H. PEARCE is the author of numerous life-changing non-fiction books for women, including: *Burning Woman; The Rainbow Way: cultivating creativity in the midst of motherhood* and *Moon Time: harness the ever-changing energy of your menstrual cycle* – all of which have been Amazon #1 bestsellers in their fields. Her girls' book, *Reaching for the Moon: a girl's guide to her cycles* is now also available in French, Spanish, Polish and Dutch.

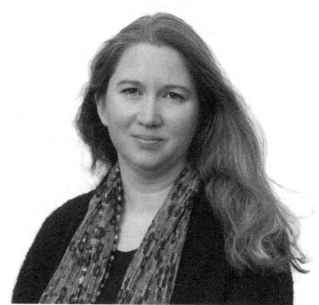

Lucy's work is dedicated to supporting women's empowered, embodied expression through her writing, teaching and art. She lives in East Cork, Ireland, where she runs Womancraft Publishing – creating life-changing, paradigm-shifting books by women, for women.

www.lucyhpearce.com

About the cover artist

ELSPETH McLEAN is a visual artist based in British Columbia, Canada. She creates her engaging, colourful and intricate artworks entirely out of dots made with acrylic paint and a paintbrush. For Elspeth, painting dots is a meditative and grounding experience.

Elspeth's love of colour and detail are how she expresses and celebrates the colours of her soul. A lover of travelling, it is the new and beautiful landscapes she explores that become subjects of her art. She has a great reverence for the seasons, cosmos, sacred geometry, the Divine Feminine and mythology that also influence her creations. She believes in the healing influences of colour and art which led her to achieving her Diploma in Art Therapy. Through her art she hopes to connect people with their inner child and to bring vibrancy and joy to their lives.

www.elspethmclean.com

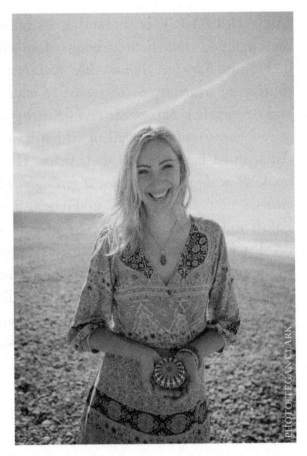

PHOTO: TEGAN CLARK

Full Circle Health
3-Month Charting Journal

Three months of blank Daily Charting and Monthly Review pages in one beautiful volume. Available now from your favourite retailer.

A download of blank Daily Charting and Monthly Review pages for home printing and personal use is also available on **shop.womancraftpublishing.com**

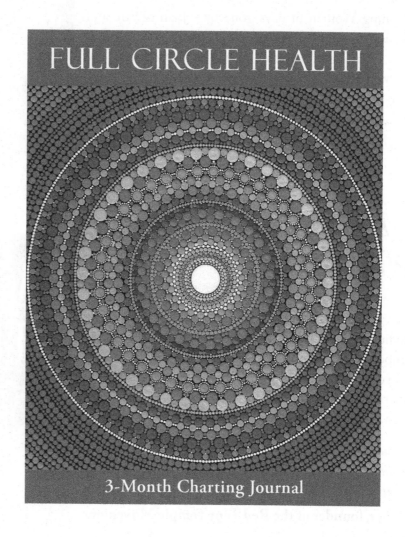

Also by Womancraft Publishing

Burning Woman
Lucy H. Pearce

A breath-taking and controversial woman's journey through history - personal and cultural - on a quest to find and free her own power.

Uncompromising and all-encompassing, Pearce uncovers the archetype of the Burning Women of days gone by - Joan of Arc and the witch trials, through to the way women are burned today in cyber bullying, acid attacks, shaming and burnout, fearlessly examining the roots of Feminine power - what it is, how it has been controlled, and why it needs to be unleashed on the world in our modern Burning Times.

A must-read for all women! A life-changing book that fills the reader with a burning passion and desire for change.

Glennie Kindred, author of *Earth Wisdom*

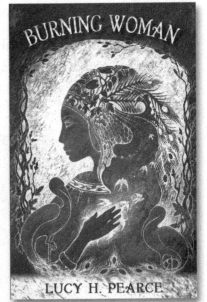

Moon Time: harness the ever-changing energy of your menstrual cycle
Lucy H. Pearce

Hailed as 'life-changing' by women around the world, *Moon Time* shares a fully embodied understanding of the menstrual cycle. Full of practical insight, empowering resources, creative activities and passion, this book will put women back in touch with their body's wisdom. Amazon #1 bestseller in Menstruation.

Now available in Spanish translation: *Tiempo de Luna* (Olinyoli)

Lucy, your book is monumental. The wisdom in Moon Time sets a new course where we glimpse a future culture reshaped by honoring our womanhood journeys one woman at a time.

ALisa Starkweather, founder of the Red Tent Temple Movement

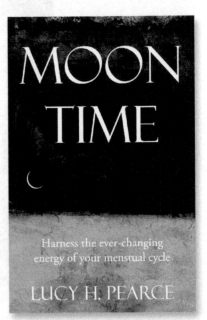

Dirty & Divine:
a transformative journey through tarot
Alice B. Grist

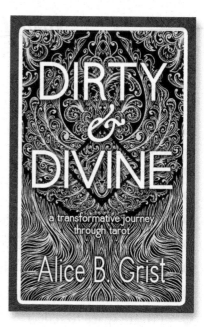

There is something sacred within you, in all that you are and all that you do. In a mix of you that is everyday dirty, and spiritually divine, there is something so perfect, something more. Welcome to your journey back home; to your dirty, divine passage back to you.

Wherever you are, whether beginner or seasoned tarot practitioner, *Dirty & Divine* is written for you, to accompany you on a powerful personal intuitive journey to plumb the depths of your existence and encompass the spectrum of wisdom that the cards can offer.

Dirty & Divine is a tarot-led vision quest to reclaiming your femininity in all its lucid and colourful depths.

Alice has been my go-to woman for tarot readings for years now, because her truth, knowledge + wisdom are the REAL DEAL.

Lisa Lister, author of *Love your Lady Landscape*

The Goddess in You
Patrícia Lemos and Ana Afonso

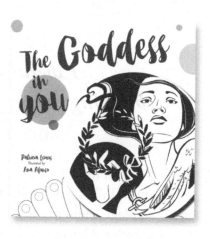

The Goddess in You is especially created for girls aged 9-14 years, offering a unique, interactive approach to establishing cycle awareness, positive health and well-being. It contains thirteen beautifully designed cycle mandalas, each illustrated with a goddess from Greek mythology.

Easy to understand and attractive to use, this powerful book celebrates what it means to be a girl growing into womanhood.

- 13 double-sided cycle mandalas illustrated with goddesses

- Instructions for use

- An introduction to the 13 featured Greek goddesses

- A basic, age-appropriate introduction to the menstrual cycle

- Self-care tips for health and well-being

A beautiful resource... Both psychologically sophisticated and delightfully simple to use, I warmly recommend this book to girls, parents and schools.

Jane Bennett, author of *A Blessing Not a Curse*

A simple and beautiful invitation to help girls build a relationship with their menstrual cycle. We highly recommend this book for all young menstruating women.

Alexandra Pope and Sjanie Hugo Wurlitzer, co-authors of *Wild Power*

Moon Dreams Diary
Starr Meneely

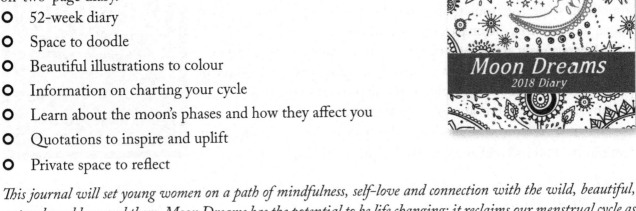

Nurturing mindfulness, reflectiveness and awareness of our body, feelings, menstrual cycle, and the cycle of the moon, *Moon Dreams* is a simple yet powerful tool in the form of a beautifully illustrated week-on-two-page diary.

- 52-week diary
- Space to doodle
- Beautiful illustrations to colour
- Information on charting your cycle
- Learn about the moon's phases and how they affect you
- Quotations to inspire and uplift
- Private space to reflect

This journal will set young women on a path of mindfulness, self-love and connection with the wild, beautiful, natural world around them. Moon Dreams has the potential to be life changing; it reclaims our menstrual cycle as a sacred, powerful experience, rather than the revolting weakness that modern society seems to view it as. Every woman needs to get her hands on one!

Lucy AitkenRead, *Lulastic and the Hippyshake*

Liberating Motherhood:
birthing the purplestockings movement
Vanessa Olorenshaw

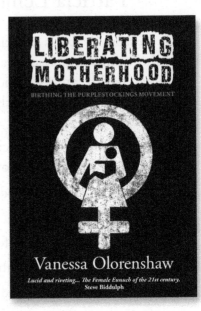

If it is true that there have been waves of feminism, then mothers' rights are the flotsam left behind on the ocean surface of patriarchy. Mothers are in bondage – and not in a 50 Shades way.

Liberating Motherhood discusses our bodies, our minds, our labour and our hearts, exploring issues from birth and breastfeeding to mental health, economics, politics, basic incomes and love and in doing so, broaches a conversation we've been avoiding for years: how do we value motherhood?

Highly acclaimed by leading parenting authors, academics and activists, with a foreword by Naomi Stadlen, founder of Mothers Talking and author of *What Mothers Do*, and *How Mothers Love*.

Lucid and riveting... This is The Female Eunuch of the 21st century.
Steve Biddulph, bestselling author of *Raising Boys, Raising Girls* **and** *The Secret of Happy Children*

Liberating Motherhood is an important contribution to a vital debate of our times. Vanessa Olorenshaw speaks with warmth, wit and clarity, representing lives and voices unheard for too long.
Shami Chakrabarti, author of *On Liberty*, **former director of Liberty and formerly "the most dangerous woman in Britain"**

The Heroines Club:
a mother-daughter empowerment circle
Melia Keeton-Digby

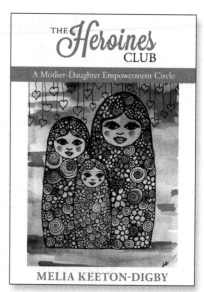

The Heroines Club offers nourishing guidance and a creative approach for mothers and daughters, aged 7+, to learn and grow together through the study of women's history. Each month focuses on a different heroine, featuring athletes, inventors, artists, and revolutionaries from around the world – including Frida Kahlo, Rosalind Franklin, Amelia Earhart, Anne Frank, Maya Angelou and Malala Yousafzai as strong role models for young girls to learn about, look up to, and be inspired by.

Offering thought-provoking discussion, powerful rituals, and engaging creative activities, *The Heroines Club* fortifies our daughters' self-esteem, invigorates mothers' spirits, and nourishes the mother-daughter relationship. In a culture that can make mothering daughters seem intimidating and isolating, it offers an antidote: a revolutionary model for empowering your daughter and strengthening your mother-daughter relationship.

The Heroines Club is truly a must-have book for mothers who wish to foster a deeper connection with their daughters. As mothers, we are our daughter's first teacher, role model, and wise counsel. This book should be in every woman's hands, and passed down from generation to generation.

Wendy Cook, founder of Mighty Girl Art

Reaching for the Moon:
a girl's guide to her cycles
Lucy H. Pearce

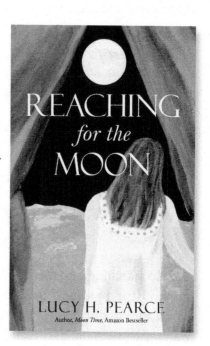

The girls' version of Lucy H. Pearce's Amazon bestselling book *Moon Time*. Written for girls aged 9–14 as they anticipate and experience their body's changes, *Reaching for the Moon* is a nurturing celebration of a girl's transformation to womanhood.

Now available in the following translations:
Reiken naar de Maan (Dutch, Womancraft Publishing)
Rejoindre la Lune (French, Womancraft Publishing)
Alcanzando la Luna (Spanish, Olinyoli)
W Rytmie Księżyca (Polish, Yemaya)

A message of wonder, empowerment, magic and beauty in the shared secrets of our femininity... written to encourage girls to embrace their transition to womanhood in a knowledgeable, supported, loving way.

thelovingparent.com

The Heart of the Labyrinth
Nicole Schwab

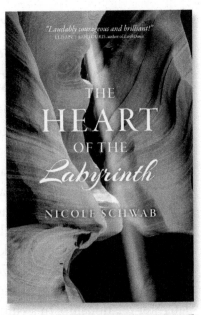

Reminiscent of Paulo Coelho's masterpiece *The Alchemist* and Lynn V. Andrew's acclaimed *Medicine Woman* series, *The Heart of the Labyrinth* is a beautifully evocative spiritual parable, filled with exotic landscapes and transformational soul lessons.

Once in a while, a book comes along that kindles the fire of our inner wisdom so profoundly, the words seem to leap off the page and go straight into our heart. If you read only one book this year, this is it.

Dean Ornish, M.D.,
President of the Preventive Medicine Research Institute,
Clinical Professor of Medicine, University of California
and author of *The Spectrum*

Moods of Motherhood:
the inner journey of mothering
Lucy H. Pearce

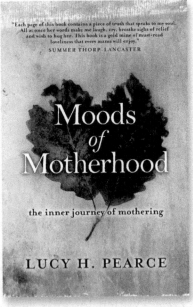

Moods of Motherhood charts the inner journey of motherhood, giving voice to the often nebulous, unspoken tumble of emotions that motherhood evokes: tenderness, frustration, joy, grief, anger, depression and love.

Lucy's frank and forthright style paired with beautiful, haunting language and her talent for storytelling will have any parent nodding, crying and laughing along — appreciating the good and the bad, the hard and the soft, the light and the dark. A must-read for any new parent.

Zoe Foster, *JUNO* magazine

The Other Side of the River:
stories of women, water and the world
Eila Kundrie Carrico

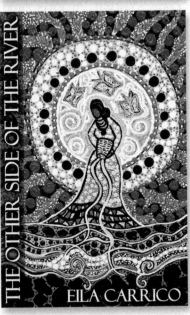

A deep searching into the ways we become dammed and how we recover fluidity. It is a journey through memory and time, personal and shared landscapes to discover the source, the flow and the deltas of women and water. Part memoir, part manifesto, part travelogue and part love letter to myth and ecology, *The Other Side of the River* is an intricately woven tale of finding your flow... and your roots.

An instant classic for the new paradigm.

Lucia Chiavola Birnbaum, award-winning author
and Professor Emeritus

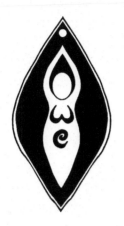

Womancraft
PUBLISHING

Life-changing, paradigm-shifting books
by women, for women

WWW.WOMANCRAFTPUBLISHING.COM

Sign up to the mailing list for discounts and see samples of
forthcoming titles before anyone else.

(f)   Womancraft Publishing

(t)   WomancraftBooks

(ig)   Womancraft_Publishing

If you have enjoyed this book, please leave a review
at your favourite retailer or Goodreads.